The Chromosome Disorders
An Introduction for Clinicians

To my friends and colleagues who have helped me so much in personal discussions, and to the many authors whose works I have pillaged without acknowledgment.

The Chromosome Disorders
An Introduction for Clinicians

G. H. Valentine, *MB ChB* (*Bristol*) *MRCP DCH FRCP(C)*

Professor of Paediatrics,
University of Western Ontario

Physician, War Memorial Children's Hospital
London, Canada

Second Edition

William Heinemann Medical Books Limited
London

First published 1966
Reprinted 1968
Translated into German 1968
Second Edition 1969

© G. H. Valentine, 1969

SBN 433 33600 5

Printed in Great Britain by The Whitefriars Press Ltd.
London and Tonbridge

Contents

Part II

THE CHROMOSOME DISEASES

Foreword

Additional chromosome abnormalities will no doubt come to light as time goes by and some of them will be correlated with definite diseases or defects. But the more common chromosome errors and the syndromes that they cause are now well established. Further, the cytological techniques for chromosome studies are well worked out. Much of human cytogenetics has therefore passed from the realm of research and can be used as an aid to clinical diagnosis. Facilities for chromosome analysis should be made available on a service basis in the laboratories of major hospitals.

This is not to say that the need for research in cytogenetics has diminished. On the contrary, it has become more imperative and will be more difficult. Methods need to be devised for recognizing small but genetically important abnormalities of chromosomes. A study of the effects of chromosome errors on enzyme systems and other aspects of biochemistry, both in the individual and in cultured cells, can reasonably be expected to give significant results. The demonstration of chromosome errors as a cause of human disease invites careful investigation of factors prejudicing normal behaviour of chromosomes during division of germ cells and the fertilized ovum. These are only a few examples of likely research trends in human cytogenetics, quite apart from the extensive chromosome studies that will go on in cancer research, virology, and so on.

Let us recognize, then, that diagnostic cytogenetics should now to a large extent be handed over to the hospital laboratory and placed on a service basis with many other cytological procedures. This current trend establishes the need for a book such as Dr Valentine has written. Human cytogenetics is a recent development. The literature includes hundreds of papers in many journals and often employs a terminology that is familiar only to the specialist in cytogenetics. Dr Valentine talks to his clinical colleagues in their own language and with a style not often found in the medical literature. The result is a highly readable as well as an informative book which deals in plain language with a speciality of importance to many clinicians.

The physician concerned with developmental anomalies will welcome the section on dermatoglyphics. Although the study of dermal patterns has a relatively long history compared with human cytogenetics, there is seldom time for teaching dermatoglyphic analysis in the crowded medical curriculum. The interpretation of dermal patterns is likely to be as mysterious to many physicians as the analysis of chromosome complements. Since both types of investigation are often carried out on the same patient, they are logically brought together in this book.

It is a pleasure to point to the happy and profitable collaboration that

ix

has gone on for several years between the Department of Anatomy and clinical departments in this Faculty of Medicine. This book is evidence enough of the good communication between paediatricians and anatomists. Of the latter group, Dr D. H. Carr, Dr H. C. Soltan, and Dr F. R. Sergovich have been especially involved in genetic and chromosome studies on patients under clinical investigation by Dr Valentine and his colleagues. Our contacts with clinicians make the work in a basic science department more interesting and rewarding than it otherwise would be.

I expect that the reader will enjoy this book and I wish it well.

MURRAY L. BARR, M.D., LL.D.

Department of Anatomy
University of Western Ontario
London, Canada

September, 1965

Preface to Second Edition

I hardly expected, when I had the temerity to write this little book, that before very long I would be writing it all again. Of course I hoped that it would be well received, but the demand for a new edition has been as surprising as it has been gratifying.

When I embarked upon the first edition it was my belief that such a naive endeavour might be justified by a need, in this age of overwhelming knowledge explosion, for what I may perhaps call "Medical journalism": reporting of a mass of new information in narrative form. It seemed to me that my best qualification for that enterprise was that I was not an expert in the field and that my knowledge was so superficial that I could not make my interpretation incomprehensible by the inclusion of obscuring details and confusing controversies. It does seem that there is indeed a place for commentary by an interested amateur.

I am sorry that the book is a little longer. It could not be helped. In 1965 human cytogenetics was very young. Three years have added to our knowledge. It would be a strange baby that showed no growth and no development. Although much of the original book remains, it has in fact been entirely re-written. The facts may not have changed in some sections, but the emphasis may have altered. On some subjects I have shifted my opinions entirely. No harm in that. It is good to be consistent; it is better to be right.

I have added considerably to Chapter I. I felt one could not dismiss the fundamentals of molecular genetics without a word. I have felt that the YY syndrome deserved detailed consideration. It is the "in-thing" of the moment. I have resisted pressures to substantiate each statement with references and a huge bibliography, not entirely because of the tedium of so doing but because I have felt that this book should be (as one reviewer kindly remarked of the first edition) information disguised as entertainment. It is not a work of scholarship. I invoke the perogative of the journalist and state that the facts I have used come from "informed sources".

Those informed sources have remained unfailingly helpful. Without their encouragement and support I could never have written either edition of this book. Their help is acknowledged in the Preface to the first edition, but I must acknowledge personal contacts with new informants. The participants at our annual "Great Lakes Chromosome Conference" have helped me greatly in giving me the opportunity of previews of unpublished works and prescient hypotheses. I have unashamedly stolen the section on Antenatal Cytogenetics from one of the participants, Professor Neil McIntyre of Cleveland. I hope he won't mind. I must also admit to stealing information on the syndrome of chromosome 18 deletion from the beautiful exhibit at the American

Academy of Pædiatrics meeting in Chicago in October 1968 by Dr J. D. Blair, also of Cleveland, Ohio. He condoned the felony by giving me the illustrations that I have used. There are, of course, innumerable informed sources whom I have never met; those who have written all the papers that I have pillaged without acknowledgment by reference. Perhaps they will be consoled by the realization that, having to be most discriminating in what I chose to include in so small a book, I plundered only those facts or conclusions that seemed of especial value.

Miss Leonie Duncan of the University of Western Ontario Medical Art Service has added new illustrations and revised some of the originals. The Cytogenetics Laboratory of Victoria Hospital have supplied some new karyotypes. My new secretary Jan Breton has laboured with unfailing good humour on the manuscript. When Helen Fisher left me to move with her husband who took a position elsewhere I was dismayed, for I was already committed to write this new edition. Jan had a grim initiation into a new job, for I started to write this book the day she came. With her came testimonials that read "No matter how much work she has to do, she is always as cheerful as a cricket. Nothing is too much trouble". How true that is.

Department of Pædiatrics
University of Western Ontario
London, Canada

January, 1969

Preface to First Edition

Nowadays one can scarcely pick up a medical journal without being confronted, confused and confounded by articles presenting pictures and diagrams in which little x-shaped bodies float like letters in a bowl of "alphabet soup" or are arrayed like rows of little dancing men. The text, with its neologisms and jargons, compounds the confusion of the average reader, and yet the multitude of these articles must surely testify to the importance of the little bodies thus portrayed. Some, of course, can read this strange writing, but perhaps to the majority it means no more than do the hieroglyphics of the Egyptians or the script of Babylon. Under the tutelage of good friends and colleagues versed in these matters I have tried to learn what these little symbols mean. I cannot understand it all, but I have come to see something of what this hieroglyphic code spells out. This book is an attempt to pass this information on in simple terms.

I am not a cytogeneticist. I am a clinical pædiatrician who deals in anything from warts to wheezes, from mumps to mongolism. I mention this so that cytogeneticists may forgive and so that my clinical colleagues may take heart. To any of the former who should happen upon this book I say: "put it down at once. Its naivety will shock you. This is not for you". To the latter I would say: "take courage; if I can understand this much, it must indeed be capable of comprehension".

This book is intended to be a narrative of our knowledge up to the present time. It is not a work of scholarship. It is for that reason that I have chosen to write in a somewhat conversational style. If at times it seems to be repetitious and perhaps verbose it is because I personally find new ideas difficult to grasp first time around. I hope my readers may feel as I do: that I would rather be encouraged by discovering that I have more perception than is expected of me than be dismayed by finding I am more stupid than the author seems to think.

The lack of references may seem to be heretical in these times when every sentence in a book of medicine must, it seems, be fragmented, and lose something of its meaning, by strings of names in parenthesis; or by rows of little numbers. This book is a story-book. It is not an exhaustive text. To assist those who would learn more of this subject I have supplied a list of those writings that I have found to be helpful, of interest and not too obscure. That the one book that is recommended above all others is produced by the publishers of this book is no more than coincidence!

This book is, of course, a work of pillage and piracy. I have taken the facts, as they seem to me, from many sources. I have no new knowledge of my own to impart. Where I have come up against controversial matters I have taken the line of least resistance, and have either adopted one point of view; or have confessed my ignorance. Those experts whose works have been purloined will, I hope, forgive my plundering, even though no individual acknowledgments are made. I must acknowledge that the whole book is the work of others; but I wrote it, and its errors are mine.

Nevertheless, I must express my especial indebtedness to some. My friends and colleagues in this university, Professor Murray Barr, Dr David Carr, Dr Hubert Soltan, Dr Earl Plunkett and Dr Fred Sergovich have helped me greatly with their discussion of my often foolish questions. They have helped me much with the photographic illustrations. Professor Barr most kindly read the manuscript to ensure that the simplifications and dogmas used in this treatment of such a complex subject are no worse than half-truths.

I have drawn very largely upon the writings of Dr Norma Ford Walker of Toronto, Dr Irene Uchida of Winnipeg, Dr Constance Clarke and Dr C. E. Ford of Harwell, England, Dr M. Fraccaro of Pavia, Italy, Dr D. G. Harnden of Edinburgh, and Professor P. E. Polani, Dr J. L. Hammerton and Dr N. D. Symonds of London, England. Without the great review of the sex chromosome anomalies by Dr Orlando Miller of New York I would have been lost indeed.

I must also express my thanks to Mrs D. M. Hutchinson who produced, or reproduced, such beautiful diagrams, drawings and tables. The cost of her work was most generously defrayed by the Victoria Hospital Trust, London, Ontario.

My chief, Professor J. C. Rathburn, has been most tolerant of my preoccupation with chromosomes, a preoccupation that developed while holding a grant, together with Professor Carol Buck of the Department of Preventive Medicine, from the Department of Health and Welfare and the Mental Health Foundation of Ontario, for research into the genetic mechanisms in mongolism.

By no means the least of my thanks must go to my secretary, Mrs Helen Fisher, who has worked so hard and so well on the manuscript. It was she who said, when the invitation to write this book arrived: "I have bad news—for both of us."

G. H. V.

Department of Pædiatrics
University of Western Ontario
London, Canada

September, 1965

Part I

THE GRAMMAR OF CYTOGENETICS

"Every problem becomes very childish when once it is explained to you. Here is an unexplained one. See what you can make of that, friend Watson."

I looked with amazement at the absurd hieroglyphics upon the paper.

"Why, Holmes, it is a child's drawing!" I cried.

"Oh, that's your idea!"

"What else should it be?"

"I think I can help you pass an hour in an interesting and profitable manner," said Holmes, drawing up his chair and spreading out in front of him the various papers upon which were recorded the antics of the dancing men.

The Dancing Men
Arthur Conan Doyle

(The hieroglyphics above spell out, in the code of the dancing men: "The Chromosome Disorders")

Chapter I

The Cell and its Chromosomes

As all mankind is believed by some to be descended from Adam and Eve, so all the cells of the body stem from that first union of sperm and ovum, the gametes, that join at conception to form the zygote. By myriads of multiplications through generations without number this first cell divides and divides again. As generation succeeds generation the cells take different developmental lines, diverse forms and functions, grouping themselves into masses and then into organs each with its special purpose to the body as a whole.

Finally the body becomes a commonwealth of organs and systems, each with its teeming population of cell citizens who contribute to the common good and receive according to their several necessities.

The health and wellbeing of this federation depends upon the correct formation of the organs as the constituent cells divide and multiply; it depends on the correct functioning of the organs as determined by the disciplined activities of the cells of which they are composed. The demands of one organ must be met by the productive efforts of another. There must be no deficiencies nor surplus. Here is the perfect common market. Would that the nations of mankind worked so harmoniously.

Not only must the body Commonwealth be constructed and set in motion, but its form and function must be preserved, even though 50 million cells die each second and 50 million are born anew to take their place. The torch must be passed from generation to generation as renewal repairs delapidation.

Here in this book we will explore a group of disorders in which it has recently been recognized that quite major and visible errors of structure of the remote ancestral cells give rise to such errors of function, passed through countless numbers of cell divisions, that in the end the development of the body is abnormal and its harmonious function is impaired. First we must consider certain aspects of structure and function of the cells about which so much has been learned since they were first recognized by Robert Hooke just three centuries ago.

The Cell

Whether it be a cell from man, fish, or frog, whether it be from liver, skin, or brain, there is a basic essential structure to a cell. Upon this basic anatomy are superimposed the differences that suit a cell to its especial function. Let us consider the essentials (Fig. 1).

There is the cell envelope which encloses its substance, but through which can pass the requirements of the cell, its wastes and its useful products.

The cytoplasm is traversed by a fine network of minute channels, the Endoplasmic Reticulum. Along these minute tubes are clustered, like berries on a vine, innumerable tiny granules, the Ribosomes. Presumably this endoplasmic reticulum network facilitates the passage within the cell of the output of the ribosomes which, as we shall see, are the work-benches on which are forged the products of cell activity.

The mitochondria are the power packs of the cell. Here is made and renewed adenosine triphosphate (ATP) the fuel of cell activity. The Golgi bodies serve as warehouses and packing stations for the cell's products.

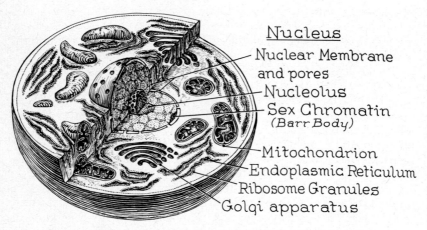

Fig. 1. Schematic drawing of a typical cell showing its main component parts. (*Adapted from The Cell, Life Science Library, Time Inc, New York*)

Somewhere within the cytoplasm lies the nucleus, contained within its perforated membrane, controlling all.

For a long time it has been known that every active living cell contains this nucleus, and that within this nucleus is to be found material that stains darkly with many stains. Except in the dividing cell this chromatin material appears at first sight as irregular shapeless masses with no pattern of arrangement. About a century ago it was observed that when a cell divides some order becomes apparent in the nucleus. The amorphous chromatin becomes condensed into a number of finite bodies, dimly recognizable in shape, in a number constant for the species whose dividing cells are under scrutiny. These are the chromosomes. These are the instructors of the cell, its government, invisible when engaged upon their business of regulation of the affairs of the active cell; visible when in recess as the cell prepares and proceeds to divide.

The Chromosomes

Each chromosome is a long long strand of deoxyribonucleic acid (DNA) which was shown by the brilliant work of Watson, Crick and Wilkins in 1953 to be in the form of a ladder. The side pieces are composed of a sugar, deoxyribose, and phosphate. The rungs are four nucleotide bases: cytosine (C), guanine (G), adenine (A), and thymine

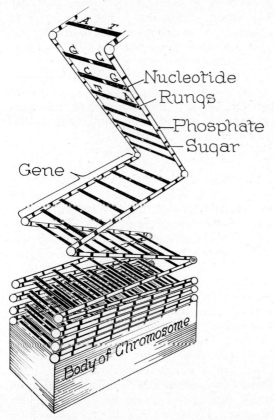

Fig. 2. Author's concept of the way in which gene links may be embodied in a chromosome and may be extended or condensed. For simplicity of illustration the ladder is drawn straight and not in the accepted helical form.

(T). It is now known that the ladder is twisted into a double helix or spiral staircase, but for the sake of simplicity of illustration we will omit that detail and consider the ladder as rather resembling the long extending ladder of a fire truck. It can be extended or it can be condensed to a pile of segments closely packed together (Fig. 2).

The rungs are each of two parts; two bases form each rung. Cytosine is joined to guanine to form one type of rung; adenine and thymine join to form the other type. These two types of rungs may be arranged spatially in the ladder to give four variants: guanine-cytosine, cytosine-guanine, adenine-thymine and thymine-adenine.

The order in which the rungs succeed one another can be infinitely varied. Thus one could have a sequence: GC, CG, AT, TA; or GC, CG, AT, AT; or GC, AT, CG, TA. Innumerable formations and combinations are possible within a ladder of just a few rungs. Fifteen rungs can be arranged in more than a billion different ways. The possibilities of arrangement and re-arrangement of the rungs in the ladders of the human chromosomes are beyond belief. Perhaps 1 and 10,000 zeros to follow it would scarcely suffice to count their numbers.

It is believed that the infinitely variable sequences of rung arrangement give the orders to the body cells as to the way in which they will be marshalled as the body develops, as to their function in the organs which they compose, as to the continuing activities of their descendents and their descendent's children. How does it work?

Genes and Gene Loci

If we take on trust for the moment the notion that the arrangement of the rungs GC(CG), TA(AT) in the long ladders of DNA dictates the total and innumerable possible activities of the cell, we can imagine that segments of the ladder (and the sequence of rungs in that segment) might be concerned with individual activities. There might be sub-division of the DNA strand so that a particular portion is concerned with one activity or product of the cell. Thus it seems to be. There seems to be one segment of sequences, a gene, concerned with each specific function. It appears that there are many segments, many units of instruction, many genes on each long strand of DNA or chromosome: perhaps fifteen or twenty thousand. As we shall see, it is now known that there are in each cell of a human body 46 chromosomes. As we shall also see, they are now known to be in pairs: 23 pairs. Of these 23 pairs, 22 are identical in both males and females and these are called "Autosomes" or "Autosomal Chromosomes". They, and the genes of which they are composed, are concerned with the innumerable bodily developments and activities that are common to both men and women. One pair, the "Sex Chromosomes" are different in males and females. The female has a matching pair of chromosomes, XX. In the male the corresponding pair do not match up. One of the male pair resembles one of the female sex chromosomes, the other is quite different and is called the Y chromosome. The female is XX, the male, XY.

We do not know much about which instruction of cell activity comes from which chromosome. We know very little about the position of particular genes or "gene loci" but we know a little.

We know that a sequence on the Y chromosome instructs certain cells of the developing foetus to form a testis which in its turn produces hormones that virilize the genitalia. There is some reason of late to suspect that other genes on the Y chromosome may instruct other body cells to function in such a way that their possessor has other attributes of maleness: tall stature, aggressive behaviour and perhaps, hairy ears.

We know that certain genes or sequences occur in the X chromosome pair. The sequence that determines the manufacture of antihaemophilic globulin is there; so is the sequence that instructs the cells of the retinae concerning colour perception and colour blindness. Present also on the X chromosome is a gene or sequence that is concerned with muscle function and for the presence or absence of whatever cell activity it is that determines whether a person will have muscular dystrophy or not. We know a little about the gene instructions located upon the chromosomes that are concerned with sex determination and we recognize certain "X-linked" or "sex-linked" genetically determined diseases.

We know nothing or almost nothing about those genetic instructions which are located on the autosomes. We cannot say where are located those genes that determine hair colour, eye colour or the sequences that condemn some men to baldness. The search is on, and there are indications that the autosomes will soon reveal their genetic secrets. There is reason to believe that a gene determining the manufacture of the plasma protein haptoglobin can be located on a particular chromosome pair, that the gene for the Duffy blood group can be located on another pair and that the gene that determines the disease Cystic Fibrosis on yet another pair. Three activities only have been located (and those but very tentatively) among the thousands of activities that determine body function. We are only just beginning to map the human chromosomes.

When we say, as we have done above, that the gene for a particular activity can be assigned to a chromosome pair, we mean that each one of the pair carries a gene or segment for that activity. In the same way as a whole chromosome has its counterpart, so every segment on that chromosome has its counterpart, its "Allele" on the other chromosome. "Homologous Chromosomes" as matching pairs are called, carry genes which together make an "allele pair".

Somewhere on one of the autosomes is a sequence concerned with eye colour. On its homologous fellow is a sequence concerned with that same affair. The two instructions may agree on what pigment is to be made by the cells of the growing eye. If there is such agreement of genes it is said that the individual is "homozygous" for that gene or instruction. But there may be disagreement.

Although two homologous segments may be concerned with the same affair there may be slight differences in the arrangement of the rungs. The alleles may be in dispute as to precisely what instruction is to be carried out. The individual will be "heterozygous" for the characteristic under consideration. If one of the disparate genes takes precedence and overrules the other, that gene is "dominant" to its "recessive" allele. If there is compromise (as usually there is) the cells will turn out an intermediate product or a mixture of two products. If a gene is unpaired, if for some reason its fellow allele is missing, the individual is "Hemizygous" for that present gene, and it of course holds undisputed sway. Let us see now how the nature of a cell product is to be determined.

The Genetic Code

Suppose we have one segment on one chromosome with a sequence of rungs thus: TA, CG, GC, CG, AT, TA, CG, AT, TA, TA, CG, and so on, we see that this does indeed look like a code. It is.

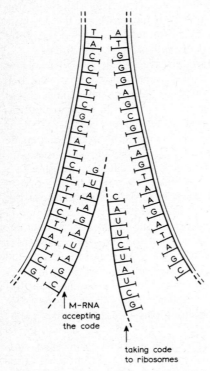

M-RNA
accepting
the code

taking code
to ribosomes

Fig. 3. Transmission of the Genetic Code. A sequence of rungs in a section of the DNA ladder of a chromosome. The rungs break apart and a strand of RNA moves in, building onto itself rungs that are the complement of those of the DNA. These M-RNA molecules move to the ribosomes where they act as the template for the construction of polypeptide chains (Fig. 4).

In the cell, busy about its everyday affairs, the ladder of sequences is enormously extended and all the chromosomes (with one exception) in long filamentous forms. Each long ladder is in a constant state of cleavage and of reforming, breakages being at the junction of the two halves of the rungs (Fig. 3). One half of the ladder now would run thus ... T, C, G, C, A, T, C, A, T, T, C, and so on; the other would run ... A, G, C, G, T, A, G, T, A, A, G, and so on.

Alongside the broken ladder a new strand of sugar and phosphate moves in: a strand of ribonucleic acid. New rungs are built on to this new RNA strand to correspond with those of the original ladder that has for a time broken away. We see in our illustrations the formation of two new half ladders. We notice also a difference from the old ladder.

In the new half ladders the reciprocal of A is not T, but another base, Uracil (U). The sequence of the old ladder C, A, T, T, C, T, A, T, C, G summons to the new RNA strand the sequence G, U, A, A, G, A, U, A, G, C. Figure 3 should make this clear.

We now have a reproduction (with the exception of the T-U change) of each half of the old ladder. These new ladders, formed on the template of the old, are the carriers of the genetic code of each chromosome to the ribosome work-benches of the cell. These are messengers: M-RNA.

Acceptance of the Code

When a protein food is digested it is split down firstly to peptones, then to polypeptides and finally to aminoacids. The proportions and variety of these aminoacids are characteristic of the proteins from which they were derived. Aminoacids absorbed into the body bathe the cells and pass into the cytoplasm where they come into close contact with the ribosomes. The aminoacids from, let us say, a beef steak bathe and enter, let us say, the cells of man.

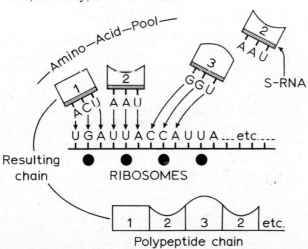

Fig. 4. Control of the arrangement of aminoacids in the synthesis of a polypeptide chain by triplet codons on the M-RNA strand. The codons attract the complementary triplets attached to the aminoacids by S-RNA. (*Adapted from Hartman and Suskind: Gene Action. Prentice-Hall, 1965*)

The messenger RNA leaves the cell nucleus and travels to groups of ribosomes. There the aminoacids have been prepared by enzyme systems and by another RNA (S-RNA or adaptor RNA) in such a way that they have an especial affinity for a particular base sequence on the M-RNA strand. Each aminoacid is attracted by a particular three-base sequence, a triplet or "Codon", because the S-RNA to which it is attached bears the reciprocal of a triplet sequence on the M-RNA strand (Fig. 4).

The triplet UUU on M-RNA attracts the aminoacid phenylalanine. Proline and Serine are attracted by the codons UUC and UCC respectively. Each of the 20 or so aminoacids has its own coded summons.

The M-RNA strand moves over the ribosomes, and as it does so the aminoacids are selected according to the sequence of triplet codons. They are selected in an order determined by M-RNA which in its turn was laid down on the template of a chromosome. Thus do the chromosomes dictate the functions of each body cell and, in the summation of cell activities, the form and function of the body: the "phenotype".

This is a simplification. Each and every cell has the potentiality of making every one of the products that is coded in its genes. All cells, be they from skin, bone, liver or from brain have the same chromosomes and the same code. In fact, of course, they do not all grow in the same way, make the same products, develop the same enzymes systems. They do not all accept all the genetic code.

In explaining differentiation of cell function we are on uncertain ground. Perhaps all one can say at this stage is that there are "Repressor" genes which call forth the synthesis of enzymes which in their turn can control the degree of transmission of the genetic code to the messenger RNA. There also seem to be proteins within the chromosome structure, histones, which are able to interfere with the transmission of some segments of the code in certain cells, and thus are able to switch on and off certain activities. Here we enter the realms of ignorance and speculation.

Gene Disorders

Apart from its intrinsic fascination, all the foregoing is relevant to our study of the chromosome disorders, for it can now clearly be seen that an upset in the sequences of DNA, an upset in the composition of a chromosome (or of the total number of chromosomes) would almost inevitably affect the form and function of the body to greater or less degree.

What has been called "classical" clinical genetics deals with minute rearrangements or confusions in the genetic code. It deals with such malfunctions as may arise when the sequence in one segment is disarrayed. It deals with minute and invisible chromosome disorders—though that is not to say that the effects may not be devastating.

For example, in the disease of Sickle Cell Anaemia there is a departure in one of the autosomes from the normal rung arrangement of both members of an allele pair that deals with the manufacture of haemoglobin. In the patient, homozygous as he is for this abnormal arrangement (both alleles abnormal), those cells that are concerned with the synthesis of haemoglobin are incorrectly instructed in such a way that an inappropriate aminoacid is summoned to the haemoglobin molecule. An abnormal haemoglobin, Haemoglobin-S is synthesized. This is a serious disease, and yet no visible abnormality can be recognized on the most careful scrutiny of all the chromosomes. Gene abnormalities cannot be seen, they are much, much too small to be resolved by any microscope.

This book deals with Chromosome Disorders, human "Clinical Cytogenetics", a term which has come to be used to describe the study of abnormalities of form and function resulting from colossal aberrations of chromosome construction or of number: Abberrations so large as to be visible even with an ordinary microscope.

It is, at first sight, odd that the science of classical human genetics, dealing as it does with minutiæ, is ninety years older than human cytogenetics, but there are reasons. The classical genetic disorders aroused interest and exhibited their hereditary and genetic nature because they appeared in members of successive generations of a family. Studies of the pedigrees of families with such disorders, together of course with the experimental work of Gregor Mendel and a century of successors, have given circumstantial evidence of the way these disorders are caused by abnormal genes. No one has seen a disordered gene, the evidence is inferential only, but is based on sound evidence derived from the descent of traits from generation to generation of plants, animals and man.

Such evidence is almost entirely lacking in the huge chromosome disorders that we consider here. Many are so disastrous that their possessor dies soon after conception, and either is re absorbed unrecognized as even a pregnancy, or is cast out as a miscarriage. Even if born alive, many babies with huge chromosome disorders are so disordered that they die in the first few days or weeks. These with disorders compatible with life are, because of the nature of their defect almost always sterile, or at the very least heavily discriminated against in reproductive opportunity. The genetically determined nature of these defects went unrecognized until just a few years ago. There was no sound circumstantial evidence. It needed the discovery of ways and means accurately to scrutinize the shape and size of human chromosomes and to determine their number before it could be realized that several disorders, long known by clinical description, were indeed genetic disorders of a massive kind. Let us look at those ways and means.

Chapter II
The Human Chromosome Complement

The Barr Body

It will be remembered that we said in our opening description of the cell that the chromatin of the active cell is in irregular amorphous masses. It will be remembered that we indicated that this was because the chromosomes were so finely attenuated that they were too thin to be seen by any microscope. In our section on the Genetic Code, however, we mentioned that there is an exception to the general rule that in the active cell all chromosomes are thinly dispersed. The exception is of great importance.

About twenty years ago, it was realized by Barr and Bertram working here in London, Canada, that one chromosome can in fact be seen

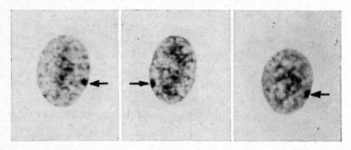

Fig. 5. Three cells showing the chromatin body (The Barr Body) alongside the nuclear membrane. One X chromosome is inactive and, in that condensed state, is visible. (*Kindly supplied by Prof. M. L. Barr*)

amidst the jumble of chromatin material even in a simple stained smear or section. On looking closely at the nucleus of any tissue of a human female, one may see in many of the cells a tiny darkly staining body alongside the nuclear membrane (Fig. 5). This chromatin mass or Barr Body, as it is often called, is not to be seen in the nuclei of normal men. This body then, in the normal human being, is a property of femaleness.

It has been known for many years that the chromosomes of men and women are identical in size and shape except in respect to one pair: that concerned with sex determination. Females possess two X chromosomes. In the jargon of the geneticist they are XX. Males possess one X chromosome and, to pair with it, a smaller chromosome, Y. Males are XY. That a man looks male, that his phenotype is male, is determined by this Y chromosome that appears to carry genes that instruct that certain of his cells should develop into testes while he is but a foetus. The embryonic testis in its turn, through hormonal stimulation, determines the differentiation and the structure of the developing genito-urinary tract. In the absence of this Y chromosome the foetal

12

testes do not develop and the body assumes the appearance, the phenotype, of a female.

It is believed that, where two X chromosomes are present within a cell, one can be regarded as spread out within the nucleus of the cell, busy about its genetic affairs, invisible. The other is believed to be largely, but not entirely, condensed and to a considerable degree inactive in transmitting its coded instructions. It is this resting and largely unrequited X chromosome that is visible as the Barr body.

Which of the two X chromosomes is active and which is genetically inert in any cell seems to be determined by chance alone at an early stage of development of the embryo, at about the sixteenth day of life. Thereafter all generations of cells will maintain the same pattern of X-inactivation as their forebears.

A female is composed of two cell populations: she is a mixture, a "Mosaic". In one type of cell one X is active while the other rests. In the other type of cell this X is resting while the other exerts its genetic influence. Most usually the two X chromosomes are so alike in genetic composition that this disparity of cell population has no demonstrable effect. But it can be otherwise.

In the female tortoise-shell cat the skin is composed of two cell populations. One area will be made of a "Clone", or group of descendants, of cells in which the active X carries the gene for black fur. Adjacent to it may be an area composed of a clone of cells which have active within them the X chromosome that determines orange hair. The black and orange brindling of this cat is the marker of the mosaicism of the cell populations of the skin.

Such disparity is less easy to detect in women, but the same effects can indeed be observed. Where a woman is heterozygous for the gene of the X-linked disorder Anhydrotic Ectodermal Dysplasia, two cell populations can be distinguished in her skin by the ability to sweat. It can be shown that one patch of skin can sweat while another cannot. In one area the X with the normal gene will be active; in the other the active X will carry the abnormal allele. Similarly in Ocular Albinism some areas of the retinæ are normal while others contain no pigment. In the woman who is heterozygous for the X-linked gene of the red cell enzyme defect 6-glucose-phosphate-dehydrogenase deficiency, two red cell populations have been observed: cells that are normal and those that have the defect.

That one X chromosome is condensed, visible or as they say, "heterophyknotic" while the other attenuated, active, "isopycnotic", is invisible was expounded as a hypothesis by Mary Lyon and bears her name as the Lyon Hypothesis.

It has become apparent over the last few years that there is not complete inactivation of one or the other X. If there were such total inactivation, an individual who had, by such mishaps as are the subject of this book, one X chromosome entirely missing, would be as normal as one who has the usual complement XX; but she is not. It now seems as though there are large zones of inactivity on one X chromosome rather than total inertia.

This partial inactivation of one X when two are present has diagnostic possibilities. A male, XY, will have no condensed and visible X as a Barr body within his cells; a normal female will have one. In cases of ambiguous genitalia and intermediate phenotype the cytogeneticist can look at a simple smear of cells rubbed from the lining of the mouth and tell us whether our patient was genetically destined, had things not gone wrong, to be a male or female. The genetic sex can quickly be determined.

If an adolescent child has not started her periods the cytogeneticist may, by looking at a buccal mucosal smear, be able to tell us that she shows no pubertal development because she has no functioning ovaries and that this has come about because one of her X chromosomes is missing. He will see no Barr body in her cells. She has only one X.

There is more to it than this. Only one X is invisible, however many may be present. If by error every body cell in a female should contain three X chromosomes, if she were XXX or triple-X, two Barr bodies would be seen. If she were XXXX, three would be seen. There is one less Barr body than there are X chromosomes. This is the N−1 rule.

In the male the same rule holds good. The normal XY male shows no Barr body, but there are males who by error are XXY. The supernumary X will retire into inactivity and will show as a Barr body. The N−1 rule holds good for both females and males alike.

Drumsticks

Another way in which the number of X chromosomes can easily be determined, though with less certainty than by buccal mucosal smear, is by examination of the lobed nuclei of the polymorph leukcocytes of the peripheral blood in a simple stained film.

It was observed by Davidson and Smith in 1954 that between 1 and 10 per cent (average 3 per cent) of the polymorphs of females have a small accessory nuclear lobule resembling a drumstick (or perhaps more closely a badminton racquet) projecting from the main mass of the nuclear lobes (Fig. 6). Such is not seen in the polymorphs of males. It seems an inescapable conclusion that this tiny lobule is composed of the condensed and heteropycnotic X of females.

Unfortunately the N−1 rule does not hold good for drumsticks when the number of X chromosomes exceeds two. Females who are XXX very rarely indeed show two drumsticks, and XXXX females never show three.

The study of the number of Barr bodies in a simple mucosal smear, and to a less helpful extent an examination for drumsticks, can tell us how many X chromosomes are present. We need only simple stains and an ordinary microscope. These simple tools will not suffice to tell us any

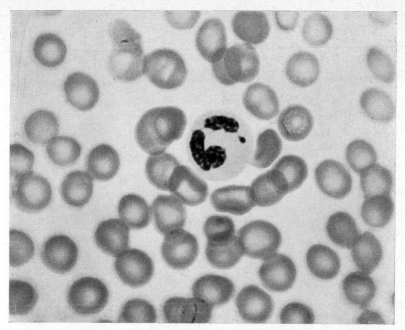

Fig. 6. Polymorph leucocyte from a female showing "drumstick" lobule. Such are found in a small proportion of polymorphs of females; they are not found in males. (*Preparation by Prof. M. L. Barr*)

more about the autosomes than can be rather dimly discerned by a study of those cells which may by chance be seen in division in a stained microscopic section. To learn more of the size, shape and exact number of all the chromosomes new and quite elaborate methods of tissue culture are required.

The Autosomes

As long ago as 1912 Von Winiwarter claimed to have observed that 47 was the normal human complement. It was nearly right. In 1923 Painter concluded that the correct number was 48 and so it was believed for the next 30 years and more.

In 1956 Tjio and Levan in Sweden used tissue cultures of foetal lungs to obtain suitable preparations of dividing cells to allow of a clear look at human chromosomes in detail. They showed, and others quickly confirmed, that the true number was in fact 46.

Very soon methods were developed for the study of other and adult tissue. Unfortunately few human tissues will grow well in culture but methods of culture of fibroblasts from skin and fascia, of cells from bone marrow and, most accessible of all, of lymphocytes from peripheral blood have been devised. Apart from their accessibility, blood lymphocytes have the advantage that a tissue culture can be completed in three days. A bone marrow culture may take a month or more; a culture of fibroblasts may be ready only after two or three months. On the other hand cultures of fibroblasts can be made many hours after death and the material can be used even after shipment by mail.

Blood cells are more delicate and do not survive more than a few hours, a day at most, of travel. There are, however, reasons apart from more robust qualities, that make it desirable sometimes to sample tissue other than blood. Sometimes the chromosome complement is not uniform throughout all body cells. More of this later.

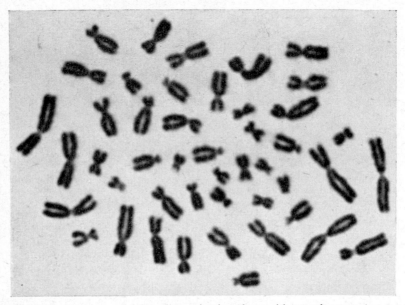

Fig. 7. Photomicrograph of a cell growing in culture with growth arrested at metaphase. Each chromosome at this stage is made up of two chromatids joined at the centromere. (*Kindly supplied by Dr D. H. Carr*)

Briefly the method of culture of blood cells is thus: A heparinized venous blood sample is taken (preferably after a few hours fast) with special precautions to ensure sterility. To this is added phytohaemagglutinin, a mucoprotein extracted from red navy beans. This has a most powerful action in stimulating the small lymphocytes to divide and multiply. The granulocytes die and disappear. The extract of beans also encourages sedimentation of the red cells which may be removed either by decanting or by very light centrifugation. The separated lymphocyte suspension is added to a culture medium with which may be included antibiotic and antifungal agents.

After three days or so of incubation Colchicine is added. This arrests cell division at a stage when the chromosomes are condensed, separated and distinctly visible, at metaphase.

A hypotonic sodium citrate solution is added after two hours of exposure to colchicine. This swells the cells and separates the chromosomes within. A drop of culture suspension may then either be placed on a slide and squashed beneath a cover slip or it may be spread as a film and dried in air. Staining and examination by the highest power of a light microscope reveals the dividing cells and their chromosomes in the form which has become only too familiar in the pages of our medical journals. What we see rather closely resembles the "Alphabet Soup" beloved of children (Fig. 7). It will be observed that there are only two kinds of "letters" in this alphabet. Some are like an X with a waist or centromere somewhere about the middle (this does not mean that they are all X chromosomes). Some are like a Y or a wishbone (this does not mean that they are all Y chromosomes). The two parts that are joined at the centromere are known as chromatids.

It must be clearly grasped at this point that these two chromatids are components of a single chromosome. One centromere, one chromosome is the rule. The chromosome is in the form of two chromatids joined at a centromere because division is (or would be, were it not for the colchicine) just about to take place. When that happens each chromatid will share half of the centromere and become a chromosome in its own right. The pieces on either side of the centromere are referred to as the "long arms" and the "short arms". In human chromosomes they are not normally of precisely the same length, though in some chromosomes they are very nearly so.

Those chromosomes in which the waist is very near the middle are known as "metacentrics", those with the centromere very close to the end as "acrocentrics"; there are those that are intermediate: "submedian" and "subterminal". They vary in size from $1 \cdot 5 \, \mu$ to $7 \, \mu$.

If a photograph, enlarged 3000–4000 times, is made of this dividing cell the chromosomes can be cut out with scissors. By trial and error they can be matched for size and for position of the centromere: long metacentric with long metacentric, large acrocentric with large acrocentric, small metacentric with small metacentric. They can be paired, and it will be found that in the human female there are 23 pairs, 46 in all. There will be 22 pairs of autosomes and a pair of medium-sized almost metacentric chromosomes XX, quite difficult to separate from a number of other medium-size submetacentrics.

In the male there will be 22 pairs of autosomes, an unpaired almost median X and a small unpaired acrocentric, Y. At first sight this Y chromosome looks like any of the other small acrocentrics, but it is subtly different. The long arms are a little longer and thinner and are usually in slightly closer apposition than is the case with the other four small acrocentrics. The female, then is 44XX, the male 44XY.

By a convention agreed upon by cytogeneticists in Denver, U.S.A. in 1960, the pairs are arranged in groups according to their length and position of centromere. These groups are designated by letters, and the individual pairs identified by number 1 to 22, plus XX or XY. This array of the chromosome complement is called the "Karyotype" (Fig. 8a, b).

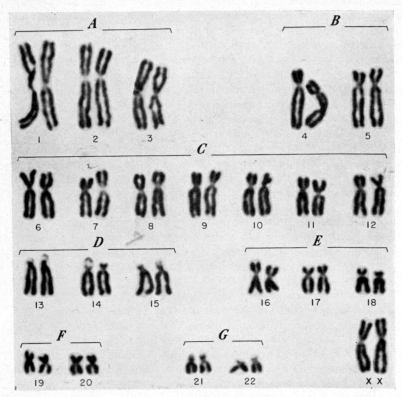

Fig. 8a. Normal Karyotype from a female showing the complement 44 + XX. The chromosomes are cut out from such a photograph as Fig. 7 and are arranged according to the 1960 Denver Convention. Note the satellites on pairs 13 and 14. These are a feature of the acrocentric chromosomes, but they are not always seen as clearly as this. (*Preparation by Dr. F. Sergovich*)

It is clear that some pairs are so similar that they cannot readily be distinguished. Chromosome 1 and its fellow are easily recognized, but who is to say, at least on fairly superficial study, which of the small acrocentrics should be paired together and which pair is to be called 21, and which 22. The certain recognition and categorization is a problem that has not yet been satisfactorily solved, but certain finer points in the appearance of some chromosomes has aided in identification. Some chromosomes have narrowed or poorly staining segments at specific points on the arms. These are called "Secondary Constrictions". They are difficult for the inexpert to see, and a very high quality of preparation and photography are required for their recognition. It is claimed by some that number 21 has a secondary constriction in its long arm, but that 22 does not. Chromosome 1 has a secondary constriction close to the centromere on the long arms; in chromosome 2 it is more toward the

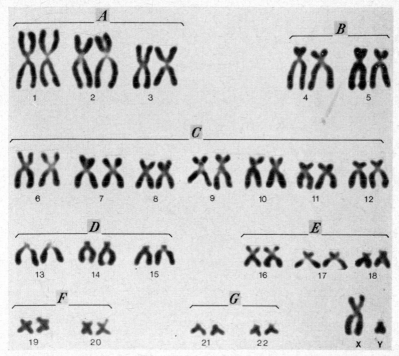

Fig. 8b. Normal karyotype from a male, XY. The length and thickness of metaphase chromosomes varies somewhat according to the preparation. Note that the satellites seen on the group D chromosomes in Fig. 8a are not seen in this karyotype. Satellites are rather inconstant features. (*Preparation by Dr F. Sergovich*)

end. The C group chromosome 6 has secondary constrictions on both long and short arms. The somewhat similar X chromosome has none at all. Sometimes on the acrocentric chromosomes there is a very long secondary constriction on the short arms so that the terminal part is separated from the rest by an almost invisible strand of poorly staining material. Such terminal knobs, beyond a long constriction, are known as satellites (Fig. 8a). An "idiogram" (a diagrammatic representation of chromosomes is so called) illustrates some secondary constrictions (Fig. 9).

By 1956 we had arrived at the point when it could be said, on the basis of a buccal smear, how many X chromosomes are present in a cell: one more than the number of Barr bodies visible. Moreover the autosomes could be seen, photographed, classified and, for the most part, identified.

While there is some variation from karyotype preparation to karyotype preparation, largely depending on details of technique, the chromosomes are remarkably constant in their sizes, shapes and numbers in the

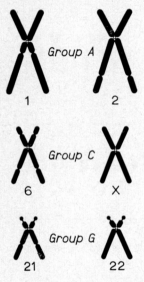

Fig. 9. Idiogram illustrating some examples of secondary constrictions. Unfortunately they rarely can be distinctly seen and are of less help in positive identification of chromosomes than this idiogram suggests.

normal individual. A departure from the normal "modal number", 46, or a real abnormality of form of any one chromosome (which must be observed in several cells) is quite unusual and, telling as it does of massive loss or gain of genetic material, is almost always associated with demonstrable disease.

To understand how chromosomes can be lost, gained, or deformed we must first look at normal cell division, for it is in that process that things can go awry.

Chapter III
Normal Cell Division

When a species reproduces sexually, a new individual commences existence when the sperm and ovum unite at the moment of conception.
These gametes unite to form a zygote. Since the zygote is the first of the
myriads of cells that by repeated divisions will make up the new
individual, mechanisms must exist for the conveyance to the gametes
individually, and thus to the zygote, of the genetic instructions that will
determine the directions of development of the new being. A genetic
code must be incorporated in this first cell, and it must be passed on
from that first cell to the countless generations to which it will give rise.

Every somatic cell of the body in a human being, be it from brain,
liver, skin or gonad, contains 46 chromosomes. Clearly, if a cell with
that constitution were to unite with another such, a zygote of 92
chromosomes would result. For the conception of a new individual with
46 chromosomes the number in sperm and ovum must be halved. This is
reduction division or "Meiosis".

Meiosis, General Considerations
Before entering into the details of meiotic division and the transfer of
the genetic code into the gametes, one must make some more general
observations. It is most relevant to note certain differences in the process
as between males and females. Let us first consider the male, for it is the
simpler.

The primitive sperm-producing cells of the testis start into meiotic
activity about puberty. Each primary spermatocyte divides by the first
meiotic division into two secondary spermatocytes. Each of these two
spermatocytes divides again in the second meiotic division, each giving
rise to two spermatids which, without further division, mature into two
sperms. A primary spermatocyte gives rise to four sperms.

This process of male gametogenesis is continuous from puberty to
death with diminishing activity with the passing years. But it is a
generous process. Sperms are made fresh, continuously in a bountiful
supply. There is little delay from commencement of gametogenesis to
maturation: maybe two months or so. The turn-over is rapid. In the
female it is otherwise.

A female is endowed with her full complement of germ cells while she
herself is still a foetus in the womb, and it is even in the foetus that female
gametogenesis commences. The oocytes prepare for the first meiotic
division even at this early age and they enter upon the early stages of the
first meiotic division, the "Prophase" of meiosis, even before birth.
From then onward they remain quiescent, waiting the long years for

their full development to gametes, their debut in ovulation and their fulfilment, perchance, in procreation.

Before each ovulation one oocyte in prophase, summoned mysteriously from its long rest of maybe fifteen or fifty years, resumes its meiotic division. Just before ovulation the first part of the process is complete. One cell takes all the substance of the primary oocyte to itself, the other becomes a mere unsubstantial nucleus, a blighted "polar body". The secondary oocyte, now shed in ovulation, begins to divide again in the second meiotic division, but this process does not reach completion without the stimulus of fertilization. Then, with a whole new life before it, it completes division into another useless polar body and into a fertile ovum with all its great potentialities. The polar body from the first division, useless though it is, divides likewise in a second meiosis forming two further polar bodies. Three polar bodies and one ovum from each primary oocyte.

Let us re-emphasize the difference. In the male gametogenesis is a brisk and bountiful affair. The two meiotic divisions occur with little delay. Meiosis in the female is much more leisurely. The prophase of the first meiotic division lasts for years: from four or five months of foetal life to the age at the shedding of that ovum.

Meiosis, Detail

In the early stages of the first meiotic division in both males and females (in adult or foetal life respectively), the chromosomes become drawn in and condensed: the stage of leptotene (Fig. 10a, A). Further condensation of the chromosomes as the genetic ladders are stacked together brings the stage of zygotene. Remember now that each of the 46 chromosomes has a partner: 22 pairs of autosomes and a pair of sex chromosomes. At zygotene (Fig. 10a, B) these pairs meet up and come to lie side by side.

Having paired, each chromosome builds on to itself a replica. There is replication, so that each chromosome now has two chromatids joined at the centromere. But it is still one chromosome. By this change we reach the stage of pachytene (Fig. 10a, C).

Later in pachytene the chromosomes become condensed and shorter still (Fig. 10a, D), while lying closely side by side. We have indicated by drawing in openline or by blocking-in that one chromosome of each pair is derived from each of the parents of this individual whose gonadal cell is now dividing to form sperm or ova. The one derived from the mother of the subject is called "Matroclinous"; that from the father, "Patroclinous".

Next comes the most important stage, the stage that indeed has led to continual variation within species, to infinitely variable combinations and arrangements of genes, to aptitude or ineptness in the struggle for existence, and to evolution by selection of those with greatest genetic

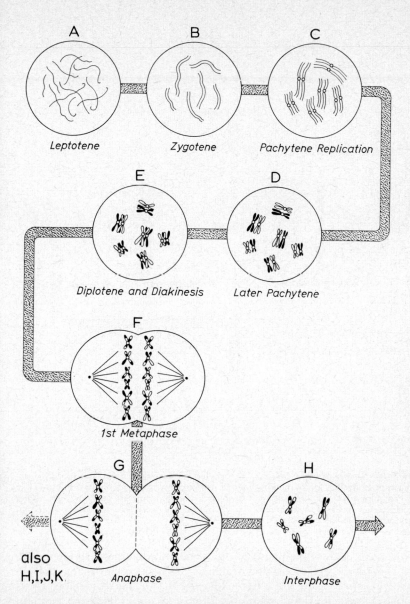

A — Leptotene

B — Zygotene

C — Pachytene Replication

E — Diplotene and Diakinesis

D — Later Pachytene

F — 1st Metaphase

G — Anaphase

also H,I,J,K

H — Interphase

Fig. 10a. First Meiotic Division. Each chromosome becomes condensed, then pairs with its homologue, then replicates becoming two chromatids joined at a centromere. Then there is exchange of genetic material with the homologue so that maternal and paternal genes are combined in one chromosome. These reconstructed chromosomes align along the line of cleavage and finally migrate into the new cell. Each cell then proceeds to a further division, Fig. 10b,

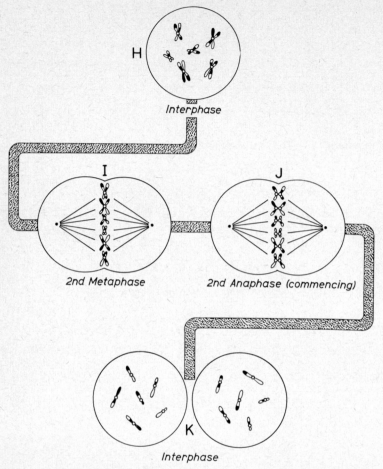

H

Interphase

I

2nd Metaphase

J

2nd Anaphase (commencing)

K

Interphase

Fig. 10b. Second Meiotic Division. The chromosomes align again, but this time the centromere divides along the long axis of the chromosome. Each chromatid now has a centromere of its own and has become a chromosome in its own right. Each gamete now has half of the number of chromosomes present in cell 10a A. A reduction division has been achieved.

advantage. This is the phase of diplotene and diakinesis (Fig. 10a, E). At this time there occurs the exchange of fragments of material from one chromosome to the other: from the matroclinous member to its patroclinous fellow, and vice versa. Breakages occur along the length of the overlapping and intertwined chromatids and there is "crossing-over" at these breakage points, known as "Chiasmata".

At the next stage, metaphase (Fig. 10a, F), we see that each chromosome is a mixture of matroclinous and patroclinous segments; each chromosome has a newly arranged array of genes, a combination never seen before, never to be seen again in uncountable years of breeding and evolution. We see also at metaphase that each chromosome aligns itself along the line of cleavage of the cells opposite to its fellow or homologue.

From the pole of each new cell filaments develop and attach to the centromeres of each chromosome. These are the spindle fibres. (Colchicine, used in the preparation of cell cultures for microscopy inhibits development of the spindles and cell division goes no further; there is arrest at metaphase).

The next process is the contraction of the spindle fibres and the "pulling", for such it seems to be, of the chromosomes into each new cell. This migration is known as "anaphase" (Fig. 10a, G). We now have two new cells formed from the gonad cell. We see that each cell now has half the number of chromosomes that was present in the gonadal cell, and we see that each of those chromosomes contains a mixture of genes: some are handed down from one lineage, some from the other.

We have now seen part of meiosis, the first meiotic division. There is more to come. Each new cell (Fig. 10a, H) has a new cycle to complete before it becomes a gamete ready perhaps to play its part in conception.

After a period of interphase, with the chromosomes each as two chromatids scattered throughout the cell (Fig. 10b, H), division starts again. The chromosomes align themselves once more along the line of cleavage (Fig. 10b, I) in the second metaphase.

Figure 10b, J shows a dramatic change. Each centromere has split longitudinally so that each chromatid now has a centromere all of its own. The chromatid is now a chromosome. One centromere, one chromosome.

Anaphase contraction of the spindles and migration of the new chromosomes into the now separating cells gives us two cells by this, the second, meiotic division. Four gametes have been produced from each gonadal cell. Each has half, the "Haploid", number of chromosomes that was present in the gonad cell which had, with its paired homologues the "Diploid" complement. Thus is reduction division (Fig. 10b, K) accomplished.

As we have mentioned, not all gametes come to fruition. In the male it is so; every gamete becomes a sperm. In the female it is otherwise. While it is true that three gametes are indeed formed, one has grown at the expense of three others, taking their cytoplasm for itself. These three cells, shrunken to mere nuclei, are useless polar bodies. There remains only one full-fledged ovum.

Mitosis

When ovum and sperm unite the diploid chromosome number, 46, is restored. Homologous chromosomes find their life partners as each brings its genetic contribution for good or ill. If the sperm brings an X

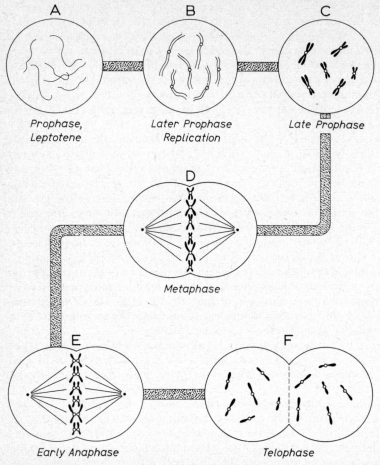

Fig. 11. Mitotic Division. The chromosomes first become condensed, then replicate, condense further and align along the line of cleavage. The centromere divides along the long axis and the long arm and the short arm of each chromatid, now having a centromere of their own, have become a chromosome. Each cell F has the same number of chromosomes as cell A. The chromosomes now become extended and commence to transmit the genetic code.

chromosome to join the X ovum, a female is conceived. A Y-bearing sperm initiates an XY male.

The zygote now divides and divides again. By myriads of divisions this cell becomes millions upon millions, yet through it all the genetic code must be preserved and pass unchanged from generation to generation. Each cell, from that first division of the zygote onward, must receive 46 chromosomes. This is mitotic division. It happens thus.

As in meiosis there is a prophase, a leptotene, in which contraction of the dispersed chromosomes commences (Fig. 11A). Later (Fig. 11B) the chromosomes are condensed, the genetic ladders more tightly stacked. Each chromosome then replicates laying down alongside itself another strand. It becomes two chromatids joined at a centromere. There is now further condensation of the chromosomes (Fig. 11C). These next align themselves along the plane of cleavage, the stage of metaphase, and the spindles develop (Fig. 11D) as in the second meiotic division. As in the second meiotic division also, the centromeres split longitudinally giving to each chromatid a centromere of its own (Fig. 11E). Anaphase migration under the influence of the spindles completes the process of chromosome segregation, telophase. The chromosomes extend, start to transmit their instructions, and each new cell is a replica of that from which it was descended.

Times without number this process is repeated so that, in the final form of the new being, each cell of every body tissue has its full complement of chromosomes: 22 plus XX or XY. Along the way these chromosomes and their genetic content exert their influences, moulding the proteins to the template of M-RNA, creating enzymes, shaping the new baby to their dictates, making a new being to a pattern which, because of crossing-over of the genes at diakinesis in meiosis, is unique; never before has there been a baby quite like this. Never again hereafter will there be another. His (or her) genes are his template for existence, his alone.

This cannot be the whole story. Not all cells are alike even though descended from a single ancestry. There is differentiation into organs of different forms and functions. In some groups of cells some genes can be "turned on" and other genes turned off. This we do not fully understand.

Even with the completion of the new being, mitosis has not done all its work. Repair of injury, regeneration and replacement of damaged and worn out cells, is by mitosis of healthy adjacent cells.

It is remarkable that such a contrivance as meiosis in two stages, union of gametes to form a zygote and growth by untold numbers of mitotic multiplications functions so well. The chromosomes meet, pair, mingle, align, retreat, unite, like dancers in a complex work of choreography. It is scarcely surprising that things can go wrong, perhaps much less rarely than we think.

Special Techniques

Although many large hospitals have established service cytogenetic laboratories there may be a need for a cytogenetic study of a patient remote from such facilities. We have mentioned that blood cells for tissue culture do not travel well. A blood sample, even if packed in ice, will grow but poorly after a day or so in transit. It may be much better, if the patient cannot travel to the specialist laboratory, to start the cells in culture—or even complete the culture process—using a "do-it-your-self" kit such as those supplied by DIFCO. If the instructions are followed carefully, a laboratory with only simple equipment can make good cultures and good slides. These can be sent to a cytogeneticist for karyotype analysis. There is even, again from DIFCO, a chromosome Micro-test Kit requiring only a few drops of whole blood from a finger prick. These kits work well.

There are occasions when one may wish to study meiosis in a human subject. The methods so far described relate to mitosis and to the array of the diploid Karyotype of 46 chromosomes. At the present time, it is not possible to study meiosis in culture and one must perform a biopsy of the gonad to study the in vivo segregation of the chromosomes.

When chromosomes are about to divide they replicate, as we have noted in our section on meiosis and mitosis. New DNA is synthesized to form the chromatids. A precursor of DNA in this synthesis is Thymidine.

The replication process is not synchronous in all the chromosomes. Some are "late replicators", some are early and some are very late. The timing of the uptake of Thymidine and its conversion to DNA varies and is, to some extent, specific for each pair. This property of asynchronous replication can help in identification of some chromosomes. Thymidine can be labelled with the isotope of Hydrogen, Tritium (H^3). It can be made radioactive as Tritiated Thymidine. If in the last few hours of tissue culture this radioactive DNA precursor is added to the medium it will be taken up by the replicating chromosomes. Their chromatids will become more or less radioactive along their length.

A squash or air-dried film of the cells, arrested in metaphase in the usual way with colchicine, is made. A well-spread cell with clear metaphase chromosomes is identified, the exact position of the slide is noted on the Vernier scale of the microscope stage. The cell is photographed.

The microscope slide is then thinly spread with photographic emulsion and allowed to stand for several days. The slide and its emulsion are then developed in the same way as is an X-ray plate. The radiations from the isotope, incorporated in the replicating chromosomes, darken the emulsion overlying the chromosomes in proportion to the extent that they have taken up thymidine from the time that it was added to the culture to the time of harvesting the cells (Fig. 12). Cells which began their replication only after the isotope was added will carry much radioactivity. Those that had started their replication earlier, those that had already used some unlabelled thymidine, will take up less. Late replicators will be most radioactive and will darken the emulsion most.

The cell, with its overlying developed emulsion is relocated and again photographed. Comparison of the plain photograph with the "Auto-radiograph" will show which of the chromosomes in metaphase are early replicators, and which are late. A pair in the B group replicates

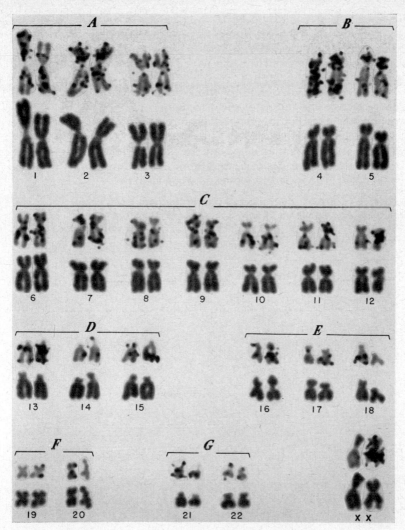

Fig. 12. *Autoradiography of chromosomes using Tritiated Thymidine to indicate the degree to which there has been replication of DNA after the addition of the radioactive precursor of DNA.* The degree of incorporation of the Tritiated Thymidine in the chromosome is indicated by the concentration of silver granules in the upper rows of the karyotype. Those that are the most radioactive are those that had taken up the least precursor before addition of radioactive precursor, i.e. the "late replicators". The X that is going to become inactivated as a Barr body is the "hottest" in this preparation. (*Preparation by Dr F. Sergovich*)

late, so does a pair in group D. In the E group 16 and 18 are slow to replicate; so is the Y chromosome. Slowest of all, and so the "hottest" of the normal chromosomes, is that X chromosome that will become largely inactive. That which would have become the Barr body can be identified by autoradiography.

I hope that the reader will not think that I have dwelt too long on genetic mechanisms and cytological techniques. Although I am a clinician I find them fascinating. But that is not my only excuse. A knowledge of the mechanisms, and of the rather unfamiliar terms used by the cytogeneticist, is essential if we are to understand the chromosome disorders. I ask the reader to bear with me a little longer only, while we discuss how cell division and segregation can go amiss.

"Let me go a little farther, a very little farther, and I will promise that you shall share everything that I know."

The Valley of Fear
Arthur Conan Doyle

Chapter IV
Abnormal Chromosome Complements

In describing abnormal chromosome complements the terms "Euploidy", and "Aneuploidy" are used. The former term describes the situation where the total number of chromosomes, while it may be abnormal, is a multiple of the total number of a normal set: in man—23 pairs. If a cell were to contain three representatives of each type of chromosome instead of the normal pair, that cell, possessing 23 × 3 chromosomes, would be "triploid". It would contain 69 in all. A "tetraploid" cell would possess double representation of each of the 23 pairs, 23 × 4 or 92 chromosomes. There can be "pentaploids" and "hexaploids". Such "Polypoidies", as they are called, presumably arise by division of the chromosomes with increase in their number without division of the cytoplasm to increase the number of cells that should accommodate them.

Certain food plants may deliberately be bred to consist of polyploid cells, with a consequent increase in size of fruit or seed, and hence a greater yield to the farmer. In the human being, with very rare exceptions, the polyploid state of the body cells as a whole is incompatible with normal foetal growth and development and with post-natal life.

The fact that the normal complement of 23 pairs, the "Diploid" number, is to be found does not mean that the chromosome complement necessarily is normal, for there may be structural departures from normal of the chromosomes themselves, without an increase or decrease in their number. We can have, then, euploid abnormalities with structural variations of the chromosomes within the normal diploid number, or we may have triploidy, tetraploidy or even hexaploidy of structurally normal chromosomes. Most, however, of the clinical chromosome anomalies with which we will be dealing in this book are of aneuploid type. The total number of chromosomes is not a multiple of 23.

Suppose that there are three representatives of one set along with 22 normal pairs, we will have a situation where a cell will contain 44 plus 3, 47 chromosomes in all. It will be aneuploid. It will be "Hyperploid", and it will be (a constantly recurring term) "trisomic" for the chromosome that appears in triplicate. Likewise single representation of what normally is a pair of chromosomes leads to "Hypoploid" aneuploidy, and "monosomy" of the chromosome that lacks its fellow. Let the reader note especially the meaning of these terms, trisomy and monosomy: three of a kind and one of a kind, respectively.

Let us look first at structural rearrangements without change in number.

31

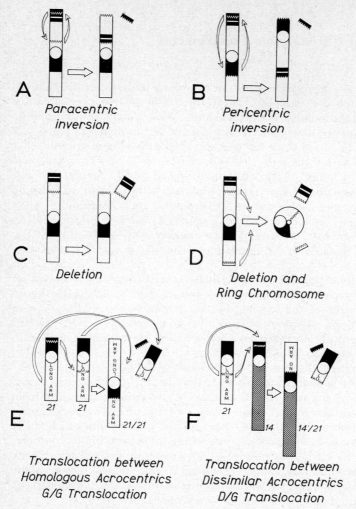

A Paracentric inversion

B Pericentric inversion

C Deletion

D Deletion and Ring Chromosome

E *21   21   21/21* Translocation between Homologous Acrocentrics G/G Translocation

F *21   14   14/21* Translocation between Dissimilar Acrocentrics D/G Translocation

Fig. 13. Chromosome Rearrangements. The rearrangements are shown as occurring in the chromosomes when they are as single strands. When the chromosomes replicate forming two chromatids, each chromatid will show the rearrangement. When part of a chromosome has been deleted as in C, the metaphase chromosome will show deletion of both chromatids in symmetrical manner. Similarly with F, both chromatids will be elongated by the translocation of additional material.

Inversion

In Fig. 13A we have drawn a single chromosome with the centromere in the middle with two bands along the length for identification. A break may occur across the chromosomes length, and the pieces may rearrange themselves in a new way. Very few genes are lost or gained, but the order in which they occur will be altered, altered in relation to the order of genes on its fellow chromosome.

Although we have no definite evidence that disease results from such a happening of itself, it may well be that such "inversions" may make for confusion at the crossing-over at diakinesis of meiosis and may also make for difficulties of the pairing of the chromosomes at metaphase—a process that is important in ensuring congruent division of the cell at anaphase (Fig. 10a, E, F, G).

An inversion that involves only one arm of a chromosome, leaving the centromere untouched scarcely alters the length of the chromosome, the position of the centromere nor, because of the imprecisions of our methods of viewing human chromosomes, even its appearance. This is "paracentric inversion".

Figure 13B shows inversion involving the centromere. The genetic load is very little changed and the length is scarcely altered, but the centromere is shifted, and with this alteration in the position of this landmark, the appearance of the chromosome has changed. In our illustration, a metacentric chromosome has become acrocentric. One can certainly imagine that such a change, a "pericentric inversion" could lead to difficulties of crossing-over and of pairing at metaphase of meiosis.

Deletion

It can happen (Fig. 13C) that a fragment of a chromosome breaks off and becomes lost; its genetic load has gone. Perhaps loss of tiny fragments and of just a few genes may permit of existence without obvious clinical effect but deletions of anything but the most minute fragments are likely to be quite harmful.

A certain man is known to the author to have one chromosome which, as a variant, has such a long attenuated constriction at one point that it amounts to a most fragile bridge between the body of the chromosome and its terminal portion. At gametogenesis this bridge broke, and the terminal fragment became lost, deleted. A child, conceived of this abnormal sperm, tiny though the missing fragment is, is quite abnormal (Fig. 63).

Sometimes it happens that a chromosome breaks so that two raw ends are left. Two tiny fragments are deleted, but the raw ends unite to form a ring, a "ring chromosome". Clinical defect results perhaps, less from the ring structure of the chromosome, than from the deletions that have occurred in its formation (Fig. 13D).

Translocation

Perhaps before proceeding we should emphasize that raw places must exist if chromosome fragments are to stick together. If a fragment breaks off a chromosome and finds no raw place to lodge, it will almost certainly be lost. A fragment without a centromere cannot survive. It can survive if it can become attached to another chromosome that, by also having suffered breakage, has a raw end. If very small, it may disappear even though it does have a centromere.

Both of a single pair can suffer a break, each losing a fragment of greater or lesser size, each being left with a raw end. The fragments may re-join in a new arrangement: "translocation to a homologue" (Fig. 13E).

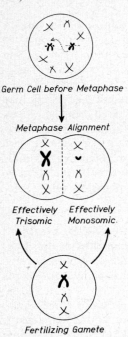

Germ Cell before Metaphase

Metaphase Alignment

Effectively   Effectively
Trisomic   Monosomic

Fertilizing Gamete

Fig. 14. Gametogenesis in balanced translocation to a homologue. In this instance it is a G/G translocation. The long arms of one G chromosome have broken from the short arms and centromere (leaving that tiny fragment) and have translocated to the short arms of the other member of the same pair (where breaks have also occurred). Two gamete possibilities and, thus, two zygote possibilities exist: one effectively trisomic, the other virtually monosomic.

While such a re-arrangement really occurs before replication and the formation of two chromatids (as in fig. 13), for simplicity and consistency with fig. 52 it is shown as happening after duplication of the arms.

One form of translocation between homologous chromosomes is that which occurs between one of the (indistinguishable) pairs in groups G (Fig. 8a, b): a G/G translocation. A tiny fragment breaks from the short arm of one of this acrocentric pair, the long arm of the other of the pair breaks close to the centromere, and two raw ends are left. The long arm from one joins to the short arm of the other and a new chromosome is formed comprising almost all the genetic material of the pair. The remaining fragment, virtually all centromere without genes, disappears from subsequent generations descended from this now abnormal cell (Fig. 13E).

But note, very little genetic material is lost, almost all remains in this translocated chromosome. Even if every body cell should be of this type—and this can happen—the person with this anomaly is normal phenotypically. They appear to be normal, they act normally, they are "balanced translocation carriers".

But (and it is a big but) gametogenesis poses great problems. When the chromosomes line up in metaphase there can be no division of this translocated chromosome. It is one and indivisible. One gamete gets all the genetic material of both of the pair; the other gets none. When fertilization brings (together with the other 22 chromosomes) one more of the pair that has undergone this homologous translocation, we have a zygote with three doses of the genetic material of this G chromosome. The zygote is, in effect, trisomic for this chromosome. The results can be clinically disastrous, as we shall later see.

If the gamete lacking the relevant chromosome is fertilized, it will be monosomic for that chromosome. That zygote will be so deprived that it will come to naught. It will not develop as a baby, nor even to the stage of a miscarried embryo. Note that each and every product of conception of a balanced carrier of a translocation between homologous pairs must be abnormal (Fig. 14). Such things can happen, and have happened.

Translocation Between Dissimilar Chromosomes

As commonly, perhaps, as between an homologous pair, there can be translocation between dissimilar chromosomes. It is true that it is usually between acrocentric chromosomes that translocations occur, but it is often between dissimilar acrocentrics; between, let us say, a large acro centric in group D and a small acrocentric in group G. For example, the entire genetic material of the long arm of one chromosome 21 may be translocated to the short arm of, let us say, one D 14. A composite chromosome, 14/21 (D/G translocation) will be formed. The centromere fragment will probably disappear (Fig. 13F).

There will be, as above, minimal loss of genetic material, and this "D/G translocation carrier" will be balanced; the phenotype will be normal.

Gametogenesis presents even more subtle problems than those explained above. Reference to Fig. 15 indicates four possible alignments at metaphase and four possible segregations at anaphase. It also indicates that four zygote possibilities exist: one with the evil effects of a triple dose of the genes of one chromosome (in this case 21), one with the even more catastrophic effect of but a single dose, one with a normal double dose by balanced translocation, and one with a normal double dose with normal chromosome arrangement. Later we will see how our knowledge of such things can guide a physician in his advice to prospective parents. I do assure the reader, yet again, that as a clinician I find these things relevant.

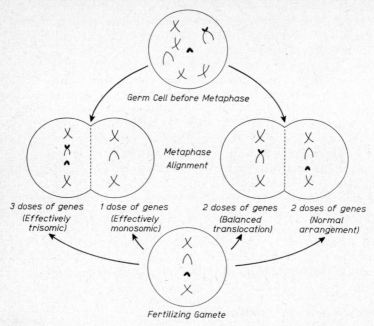

Fig. 15. Gametogenesis in balanced translocation-carrier. In this instance we illustrate a small acrocentric translocated on to a large acrocentric: a D/G translocation. It could be, for example, a 14/21 translocation. For simplicity only four pairs of chromosomes are shown. Four gamete possibilities exist. Four zygote possibilities can arise at fertilization: one trisomy, one monosomy, one balanced translocation-carrier and one with normal chromosome complement.

Isochromosomes

As we have seen in Fig. 10b, J and Fig. 11, D, E, a chromosome represented in metaphase as two chromatids joined at the centromere becomes, at anaphase, two chromosomes by division of the centromere in a plane along the longitudinal axis of the chromosome. There can be errors in this division of the centromere.

Fig. 16A shows the normal division. In Fig. 16B we see the centromere dividing, not longitudinally, but transversely. We have two new chromosomes formed, but the one will be formed of both the long arms; the other of both short arms. We can see that such an error of division would produce a giant chromosome and one that is much smaller than normal. Both would be exactly metacentric. These abnormal chromosomes are known as "isochromosome of the long arms" and "isochromosome of the short arms". Cells incorporating an isochromosome of the long arms would have the genetic content of the long arm in duplicate, but would lack the genes of the short arms. Cells incorporating an isochromosome of the short arms, while overdosed with the genes of those short arms, would lack the genetic content of the long arms. In practice this can lead to genetic imbalance and is one way in which certain of the diseases described later in this book can come about.

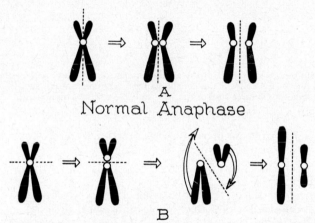

Normal Anaphase

Formation of Abnormal Isochromosomes

Fig. 16. *Isochromosome Formation.* In B the division of the centromere across the axis of the chromosome causes both long arms to migrate to one cell and both short arms to move to the other. The gene content of both cells will be unbalanced. The number of chromosomes in each cell will not be altered.

Anaphase Lag

We must now consider how a whole chromosome can be lost or gained by errors of migration of the chromosomes at the anaphase of cell division at either of the meiotic divisions of gametogenesis or at a mitotic division in the growth and development of the zygote.

In Fig. 17A, chromosomes are shown, as an example, at metaphase of the first meiotic division, paired and about to migrate as the cell divides. Should one be insecurely attached to its spindle it might "fall out" and thus be lost entirely (Fig. 17B).

Loss of a whole chromosome and its genetic content would have most serious consequences. The loss would be perpetuated in any descendants of that cell, from generation of cells to generation. An individual formed of cells from such a defective ancestry would show grave clinical effects. Indeed, loss of an autosomal chromosome in its entirety is, with one unique reported exception, incompatible with life in man. Loss of a sex

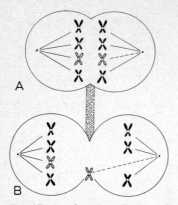

Fig. 17. Anaphase Lag. Faulty migration of the chromosomes at anaphase may lead to one being lost to one of the cells. If the cell be gamete, fertilization will supply one of the pair. The zygote will have one of the pair only. It will be "monosomic" for the pair in question.

chromosome, though permitting life, leaves the individual sterile, as we shall see.

Primary Non-Disjunction

Chromosomes, then, can be lost by anaphase lag. They can be both lost and gained by non-disjunction. Imagine the chromosomes, again in, let us say, metaphase of the first meiotic division (Fig. 18A). It can come about that a pair can become linked together so that they can migrate as one at anaphase. In the two new cells thus formed there will be an unequal number of chromosomes. One cell will have both of the pair; the other neither (Fig. 18B). This abnormal division of a normal cell is known as "primary non-disjunction".

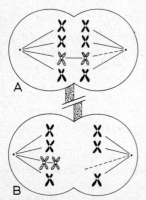

Fig. 18. Primary non-disjunction. At anaphase the two homologous chromosomes move as one. One cell lacks any representation of the pair, the other has both members. Fertilization of such gametes will result in monosomic and trisomic zygotes.

Suppose a normal gonad cell with 46 chromosomes divides unequally in this way at meiosis, the first meiotic division will yield two cells: one with 24 chromosomes, the other with 22. The second meiotic division will yield from each of these two cells, two gametes: two with 24 chromosomes and two with 22. It is irrelevant that three of the four will be polar bodies.

Remember now that each of the gametes with 24 chromosomes has both of the deviant pair represented, each of the gametes with 22 chromosomes has no representative. What now would happen if these abnormal gametes were to be fertilized by gametes of normal descent, with 23 chromosomes, each of which represents half of a pair? Zygotes could be formed with 24 plus 23, or with 22 plus 23. Zygotes of 47 and of 45 chromosomes. These would be aneuploid zygotes. One would contain three chromosomes of one kind: it would be trisomic for this non-disjunction pair. The other zygote will have but one chromosome, that brought by the normal gamete. It will be monosomic for that chromosome.

Secondary Non-Disjunction

But suppose a gonad cell should itself be trisomic because the parent individual had resulted from fertilization of an abnormal gamete; what

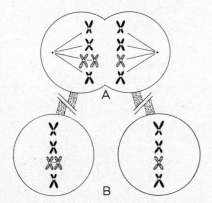

Fig. 19. Secondary Non-disjunction. When a trisomic cell divides, the two cells formed will be dissimilar. One will have two of the trio, the other one. If A is a gonadal cell and B are gametes, the zygotes will be either normal or trisomic. A trisomic parent will have (in theory at any rate) equal numbers of normal and trisomic offspring.

then? Figure 19 shows that one cell will have two representatives of the trisomic chromosome; the other cell will have one. In the second mitotic division the error would be perpetuated. Of the four gametes formed (neglecting the irrelevance of polar bodies) two will have a chromosome too many; two will be normal.

Fertilization by a normal gamete will result on the one hand in a trisomic zygote, on the other in a normal zygote. Both types of zygote would appear, in theory at any rate, in equal numbers. If a trisomic individual should be fertile such could happen. Indeed it has happened, though rather rarely.

Non-Disjunction at both Meiotic Divisions

Suppose, again, a normal gonad cell of 46 chromosomes dividing un-equally at the first meiosis (Fig. 20B$_1$, B$_2$). We will have cells with 24 and

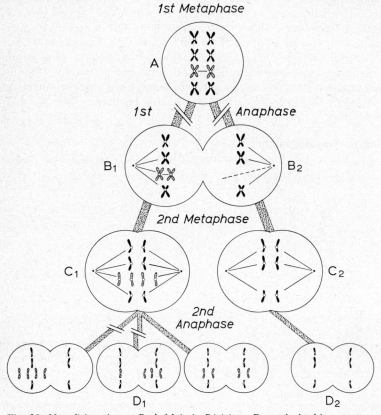

Fig. 20. Non-disjunction at Both Meiotic Divisions. By such double non-disjunction at gametogenesis, gametes can be formed that have four, three, two, one or no representative of a chromosome pair.

with 22 chromosomes. As they prepare for the second meiotic division we will see two different metaphase patterns (Fig. 20C$_1$, C$_2$). The cell with the chromosome missing will divide equally giving two monosomic gametes (Fig. 20D$_2$).

If the metaphase cell C2 should undergo a further non-disjunction at the second meiotic anaphase, we can see that a variety of gametes could be produced. There could be a gamete with four representatives of the relevant chromosome: a tetrasomic gamete. There could be trisomic, disomic and monosomic gametes (Fig. 20D$_1$).

Fertilization, of course, would add another chromosome of relevant type. A zygote could acquire five of a kind. We could have a "Pentasomy". Some such mechanism as we have outlined above may be responsible for such bizarre cases as that recently seen by the author. A girl who has a chromosome complement thus: 22 plus XXXXX, a pentasomy of the X chromosome.

Mosaicism

What about non-disjunction of the zygote at its mitotic divisions. What might this produce? Suppose a normal zygote should make an error of non-disjunction at its first division (Fig. 21A). Two abnormal cells would result: the one with 45 chromosomes, the other with 47. From then on repeated divisions might be expected to perpetuate the errors, and from these two aneuploid cells there might arise two families or clones of cells with different, and abnormal, complements. The body would be formed of two stem-lines, some bearing 45 chromosomes, some 47. The new individual, if the genetic upset were not so severe as to be lethal, would be a mixture of two dissimilar cell populations. They would be a "Mosaic" of monosomic and trisomic cells.

In fact monosomic cell lines tend to die out, and mosaicism, when discovered, is almost always of an abnormal population along with a population of normal cells. How does this happen? It may be thus.

If the first mitotic division of the zygote were to be safely accomplished (Fig. 21B), there would be, from this first division, two cells with the normal complement of chromosomes: 46. Then let us suppose that one of those cells now undergoes non-disjunction. We could have three types of cells: normal with 46, trisomic with 47, and monosomic with 45. At this point, a triple-stem-line mosaic. If, as is usual, the monosomic line dies out, we could have a zygote composed of two stem lines, normal and trisomic: a normal/trisomic mosaic.

The frequency of occurrence of cells derived in this way—the degree of mosaicism—depends on just how far development of the embryo has gone before mitotic error occurs. Error at the first division leads to two abnormal cells. Assuming that their descendants should all survive and multiply equally well (unlikely, as we have seen) the body cells of the embryo, foetus, and the child would have mosaicism of 50 per cent of each stem line.

But suppose a hundred, maybe a thousand, normal divisions preceeded an error of mitosis, the number of normal cells could so outnumber the aneuploids that the mosaicism could well be inapparent as a clinical effect. It is not inconceivable that we are all of us mosaics of some degree.

The decision for the cytogeneticist as to whether a patient from whom a culture has been made is a mosaic is not always easy. If, in a culture from a normal person, the chromosomes of 100 cells are counted it will be found that most of the cells have the same number of chromosomes. There will be a "modal" number, but some will have one or two chromosomes more than that number, some will have less. Are we dealing with

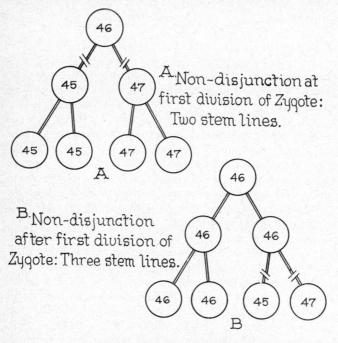

Mosaic Formation

Fig. 21. Mosaic Formation. If there is an error of chromosome segregation at the first division of the zygote, two stem lines will be formed. If the error is at a later division, three stem lines will arise. (*After D. G. Harnden, Chromosomes in Medicine, Heinemann Medical Books Ltd.*)

mosaicism, or are we looking at broken normal cells from which a chromosome or two have become lost—to lie perhaps among the chromosomes of another normal cell?

If departure from the modal number is to be regarded as something more than artifactual, it must be established that in the "Hypomodal" or "Hypermodal" cells it is the same chromosome that is missing or in excess. Moreover, if the clinical condition of the patient is consistent with the possibility of there being an abnormal stem line present, the possibility may become a virtual certainty. One must also take into account the age of the patient. Non-modal cells are found with greater frequency in cultures taken from the elderly.

In mosaicism the proportion of modal and non-modal cells may vary from one body tissue to another. It might be that every tissue sampled and cultured might show the same degree of mosaicism, or it might be that only one tissue would show an abnormality while another tissue might be quite normal. For example, a male patient has been described who showed no abnormality in culture of blood lymphocytes, yet a culture of skin fibroblasts showed the triple stem line mosaic: XO/XX/XY.

There being this possible variation from tissue to tissue, and there being the possibility of difference in chromosome complement between cells of even the same type of tissue from different sites, one cannot ever say (unless every last body cell were to be sampled) that a person may not be a mosaic somewhere, of some degree. It may be possible to say that a person is indeed a mosaic; we can never be sure that he is not.

Instability of Chromosome Complement

Having mentioned that monosomic stem lines may become extinct, one naturally wonders if changes in chromosome complement may occur from that present in the very early stages of embryonic development. This very well may happen.

Phenotypic males are known who have an apparently uniform XX chromosome complement. At first sight this would appear to negate the concept that the Y chromosome is the arbiter of testis development and of male phenotype. One such case on re-evaluation was found to have a very, very few XY cells present: (1 per cent of cells from blood culture, none in fibroblast culture). It is postulated that in this case, and the case of other apparently uniformly XX males, a Y containing chromosome complement existed as a mosaicism at an early stage of embryonic development and that the Y-containing stem line died out—or very nearly so.

This author knows of an unpublished case of a male infant whose unusual appearance and low set ears at birth led to a blood lymphocyte culture being taken at a few days of age. A ring chromosome of a C group chromosome was found in a majority of cells. There was no doubt of this. To the surprise of us all he developed quite normally both physically and mentally. At two years of age no ring chromosome could be found in any cells cultured from blood or from skin fibroblasts. His karyotype was normal! Was the ring chromosome a cultural artifact? Possible but quite unlikely. Moreover the culture was done in the first place because he looked abnormal.

How many cases of mental retardation and malformation, one asks, may have been due to a mosaicism from which an abnormal stem line became extinct, but only after irrevocable developmental damage had been done. There may be more in the chromosome disorders than ever meets the eye.

Chimaerism

This is mentioned here merely to be dismissed. Chimaerism is not mosaicism. A chimaera is an individual who has gained a stem line of cells other than his own from another zygote. Occasionally blood cell precursors of non-identical twins may interchange across the placenta in utero. Two cell lines may become established in one individual. Two strains of blood cells may result.

A chimaera has been reported where XY male cells, transfused into a newborn female baby, XX, established themselves and perpetuated a new stem line. A blood lymphocyte culture grew a mixture of cells: XX/XY. But this was not mosaicism. Mosaicism must stem from a single zygote.

At last we have finished with the grammar of cytogenetics and can turn to the clinical aspects of our subject. It is as well, I believe, to have this knowledge and its jargon behind us at this point, for we can now proceed to clinical considerations without the necessity of stopping too much along the way for explanations of unfamiliar terms.

Part II

THE CHROMOSOME DISEASES

Chapter V
Dermal Ridge Patterns, Dermatoglyphics

Before describing in some detail the clinical manifestations of the disorders associated with chromosomal abnormalities we may usefully consider a form of clinical examination that is as yet not usually mentioned in standard texts. This is a study of the dermal ridge patterns of the skin of the areas adapted for firm contact or fine tactile discrimination: the finger tips, the palms and the soles of the feet.

These ridge patterns, first described in 1684 by Nehemiah Grew and first classified by the great Francis Galton in 1892, are separate and distinct from the coarser folds and creases known to the fortune-teller. A study of the ridge patterns or dermatoglyphics (skin engravings) first aroused interest when it was noted by Cummins in 1939 that the patterns of ridges found in mongolism or Down's Syndrome—now recognized as chromosome disorder—differ from those found normally.

Digital Patterns

If you look at your finger tip with a lens (an electric auriscope with the snout removed, or an ophthalmoscope, with a +15 or +20 lens, is a good tool for such inspection) you see, as is well known, a pattern of fine ridges along the crests of which open the minute sweat pores. Presumably these ridges and the patterns that they make are to give increased friction in grasping and to give greater sensitivity of touch. (The new-world monkeys have such dermatoglyphics on their prehensile tails.) The patterns of these ridges are genetically determined, almost certainly, by the interaction of several genes.

A permanent record of ridge patterns can be made in several ways. An excellent method is to use the material marketed by Hollister Inc., of 211 East Chicago Ave., Chicago, Illinois, U.S.A. and of 160 Bay Street, Toronto, Canada. The most reliable and sophisticated method uses disposable pre-linked plastic slabs against which the area under study is gently pressed to pick up the black pigment. The digit, or other part, is again gently and evenly applied to a glossy cast-coat paper. Such pre-inked slabs retail at about 15 c. each. Alternatively Hollister market a special pad which can be used with similar shiny paper repeatedly for many imprints. Less good, but acceptable prints, can be made using an office rubber-stamp pad and a highly glossed paper. Even ordinary ink can be used provided it is not applied too thickly.

Whether you look at your finger directly or at a print you will notice that on most of the patterns there will be one or more points where a tiny triangle is formed by three rows of ridges meeting together (Fig. 22). Such a meeting point of three ridge systems is known as a "triradius".

The patterns themselves, for our purpose of clinical study, are of three varieties. There may be simply an arch-shaped arrangement of ridges bowed to a greater or less degree towards the tip (Fig. 23). In such an arch pattern there is no triradius, only an arrangement of curving parallel ridges.

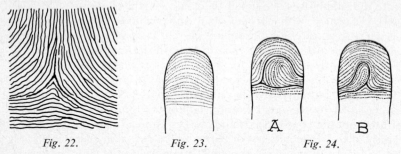

Fig. 22.	*Fig. 23.*	*Fig. 24.*

Fig. 22. Triradius. The meeting-place of three dermal ridge systems.
Fig. 23. Digital Arch. This a wide arch, as opposed to that illustrated in Fig. 27. Note that there are no triradii in an arch pattern.
Fig. 24. Digital Loops. Pattern A is a wide loop, B is narrow. The size of the loop is determined by the ridge count, Fig. 29. A loop has a single triradius. If these were on the right hand, A would be a radial loop; B would be an ulnar loop.

A much more common formation is the loop, open to one side of the digit, with a single triradius towards the opposite side (Fig. 24). A digital pattern with one triradius only is by convention a loop, though the configurations of the loop may vary considerably. There are wide open loops (Fig. 24A) and tight narrow loops (Fig. 24B). If the loop is

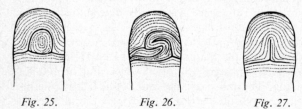

Fig. 25.	*Fig. 26.*	*Fig. 27.*

Fig. 25. True Digital Whorl. The central area is totally enclosed. Note that there are two triradii.
Fig. 26. Digital Whorl of Twin Loops. Since there are two triradii, this pattern is counted as a whorl in scoring digital patterns.
Fig. 27. Tented Arch. This narrow arch appears to have a triradius, but really only two ridge systems are involved at this meeting-place.

open to the ulnar side of the digit, that is to say the side nearest to the little finger, it is an "ulnar loop". A "radial loop" opens to the side nearest to the thumb. One triradius on a digit means a loop, ulnar or radial.

The third variety of pattern that may be encountered is the "whorl"

(Fig. 25). The typical whorl is usually formed by a series of parallel concentric ridges, but it may be formed by a spiral. In the whorl there are two triradii. Sometimes the whorl is not so clear-cut and may appear as two loops intertwined (Fig. 26), but for our purpose here a whorl is any digital pattern with two triradii.

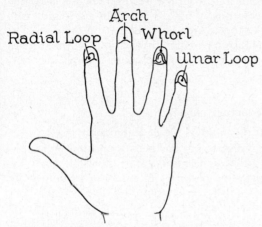

Fig. 28. The convention that is used in medical writings to indicate the patterns. The ridges meeting at the triradii (if any) only are drawn, giving a skeleton outline of the pattern. Arches are indicated by a single line.

Arches, then, have no triradius, loops have one, whorls have two. Occasionally one comes upon a loop where the centre or core is formed by one radiant of a triradius (Fig. 27). This is a "tented arch". For our purpose it is an arch.

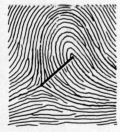

Fig. 29. The ridge count is determined by counting the ridges intersected by a line drawn from the core of the pattern to the triradius. In the case of a whorl there will be two ridge counts, one to each triradius.

Ridge lines do not always make a definite pattern. Sometimes a ridged area of skin may bear parallel lines only which form no definite arch, loop or whorl. These are "open fields".

It is customary in the illustrations in the literature on cytogenetics to simplify the ridge patterns by a convention. The three ridge lines that meet at the triradii, if any, only are drawn and followed around the pattern. A skeleton outline is given, as in Fig. 28.

Of late there has been increasing interest in the size of patterns; that is to say is it a large wide loop or a small one? Is it a little whorl or a big one? The very centre point of the loop or whorl, the core, is located and a line is drawn to the triradius. Where two triradii are found, as in a whorl, the line is drawn to that which is farthest from the core. The number of ridges crossed by this line is the "ridge count" of that formation (Fig. 29). Arches of course have no ridge count though they may be either wide or tented.

Practical Application of Dermatoglyphics

What is the purpose of all this study of such minutiae of body form? How is it relevant to clinical disease? It has been found that in normal individuals some patterns are more common than others. If one takes the patterns of both digits, ten patterns in all, and examines the frequency of occurrence of the four basic patterns, one will find that loops, both radial and ulnar, constitute 70 per cent of the patterns, whorls 25 per cent and arches 5 per cent. Ulnar loops are eleven times more common than radial loops, while wide arches are seven times more common than narrow tented arches.

The frequencies and ratios, as given above, do not hold good for all the digits individually. Each digit has its own individual frequency of patterns which in sum make up the percentages given above. For example, while on every digit loops are normally the most abundant pattern, their frequencies range from 85 per cent on digit V to 34 per cent on digit II. Whorls, while less commonly found than loops, are found more commonly on digits IV (42 per cent) and digits I (35 per cent) than on digits III and V (18 per cent and 13 per cent respectively).

There is, moreover, a difference in the two hands; while whorls are, as we have said, more likely to occur on digit I, they are more common on digit I of the right hand than digit I of the left hand (39 per cent and 31 per cent respectively). We can cite, as another example, the incidence of radial loops on digit IV where radial loops are quite uncommon, constituting only about 0·6 per cent of the patterns of both digits IV taken together. On the left hand the incidence is 0·9 per cent, on the right only one third of that, 0·3 per cent.

From a study of large populations, tables have been constructed giving frequencies of the patterns, loops (radial and ulnar), whorls and arches on the separate digits of each hand in normal persons (Table 1). Tables of normal values derived from the study of one racial or ethnic group are not quite applicable to all races of mankind. There are differences in the frequencies, though not very great, between let us say,

Caucasians and Negroes and between the Latin and Nordic strains of men.

The purpose of this compilation of data becomes apparent now that it has been realized that certain disorders that interfere with normal foetal development, and the chromosome disorders in particular, are associated with departures from the expected normal frequencies of distribution of the patterns.

Although such alterations are best known in mongolism or Down's syndrome—and were recognized about thirty years ago by Cummins—several other disorders are now known to be associated with altered

Table 1

PATTERN	I		II		III		IV		V	
	L	R	L	R	L	R	L	R	L	R
Whorl	30·8	38·6	33·4	35·7	17·4	19·4	36·9	46·6	12·0	14·6
Ulnar Loop	62·7	57·3	36·3	31·1	71·4	70·9	60·2	52·0	85·4	84·0
Radial Loop	0·8	0·8	19·4	20·3	2·6	3·4	0·9	0·3	0·1	0·3
Arch	5·8	3·3	10·9	12·9	8·6	6·3	3·0	1·1	2·6	1·1

DIGITS OF LEFT AND RIGHT HANDS

Percentage frequencies of the four basic digital patterns in normal Caucasians. (*Norma Ford Walker, Pediat. Clin. N. Amer. May 1958, W. B. Saunders Co, Philadelphia*)

frequencies of patterns so constantly that a strong indication of a particular disease may be given. Let us look at mongolism and see how an index of probability of that diagnosis can be worked out from the dermal ridge patterns of just one digit.

Table 2 shows the pattern distribution on the left digit II, the forefinger, of normal persons and of mongolian mental defectives with the disorder of trisomy of chromosome 21. One is about eight times more likely to find a radial loop on the index finger of a normal person than on that of a mongolian defective. One is more likely, by two and one quarter times, to find an ulnar loop in a mongol than in a normal person. To put it another way, the discovery of a radial loop on the forefinger of an individual makes it eight times more likely that he is normal than a mongol.

An index of probability or improbability can be worked out for each digit if the distribution of patterns in normals and mongols is known for each digit of both hands. The ultimate probability, the "digital index", is the mathematical product of the individual probabilities derived from each digit separately. The digital patterns, then, have added a measure of numerical precision to clinical impression in the diagnosis of mongolism, and to a less well authenticated extent in the diagnosis of certain other abnormalities. We will return to this subject in greater detail later in the book.

Table 2

PATTERN	DIGIT II, LEFT HAND	
	Mongol	Normal
Whorl	11·9	33·4
Ulnar Loop	82·4	36·3
Radial Loop	2·3	19·4
Arch	3·4	10·9

Percentage frequencies of patterns on the second digit of the left hand in mongols and normals. (*Norma Ford Walker, Pediat. Clin. N. Amer. May 1958, W. B. Saunders Co, Philadelphia*)

Pattern Size and Ridge Counts

The sizes of patterns as judged by the ridge counts has of late become interesting for it has been observed that the "total ridge count", that is to say the total number of ridges crossed by a line from the core to the triradius of all ten digital patterns, bears a relationship to the number and quality of the sex chromosomes possessed by an individual. It seems as though the more sex chromosome material that an individual possesses, the smaller will be the average size of pattern and the smaller the ridge count. X chromosomes seem to effect a greater depression of ridge count than Y chromosomes. The average ridge count in normal males is 145; in normal females 128, for all digits combined.

In the situation where a sex chromosome has become lost, deleted, and the individual is monosomic for the X chromosome (or is X0), the total ridge count may be raised to about 180. When, however, an individual is trisomic for the X chromosome, and is XXX, the ridge count may be about 120. If there should be three sex chromosomes, but the constitution XXY, the count may be a little higher say 130. In the sex chromosome tetrasomy XXXX, ridge counts of 75 have been observed. In the pentasomy XXXXY, as few as 60 ridges may be counted. This variation of ridge count with sex chromosome complement is not easy to explain since it is believed that pattern size is determined by genes on the autosomal chromosomes. An ingenious explanation, with perhaps some basis for its support, is that the number of sex chromosomes determines the degree of hydration of the developing foetus and the degree of oedematous swelling or otherwise of the extremities at the time when the ridges are developing, at the fourteenth week of gestation. Certainly the X0 state can lead to œdema of the extremities.

It is not only the chromosome anomalies that can lead to a change in distribution of digital patterns. Rubella contracted by the foetus from the mother in the first trimester or so of pregnancy has been shown to increase the number of whorls; only 7 per cent of normal persons have 8 or more whorls on their 10 digits. Four times as many, 28 per cent, of those who had intra-uterine rubella have more than eight whorls.

Palmar Patterns

If you now look closely at the palm of your hand you will see a number of points where three ridge systems meet in triradii. There will be one,

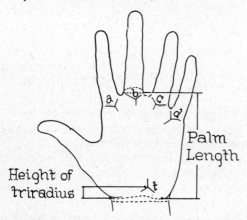

Fig. 30. The Height of Axis Triradius. This may be given as a percentage of the total palm length as measured from the bracelet crease to the middle metacarpo-phalangeal crease. Normal: less than 40 per cent.

known as a, at the base of digit II (the index finger) in the region of the metacarpal head. Similarly there will be triradii, b, c and d at the base of digits III, IV and V. There is no triradius over the metacarpal head of the thumb, but a more or less centrally situated "axis triradius" is to be found most usually quite close to the distal wrist crease or "bracelet crease" (Fig. 30). Occasionally more than one axis triradius is present, in which case the more distal is relevant to clinical analysis.

The position of the axis triradius can be described in one of two ways. The position can be stated as a percentage of the total palm length as measured from the distal wrist crease to the crease at the base of the middle finger. A value of less than 14 per cent is considered to be "proximal", from 14 to 40 per cent "intermediate" and over 40 per cent "distal"; these values are sometimes signified as t, t' and t" respectively. Alternatively the position of the axis triradius may be indicated by the angle formed by the joining of the metacarpal triradii a and d to the axis triradius, wherever it may be located: the "atd angle" (Fig. 31).

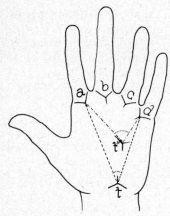

Fig. 31. The position of axis triradius may be indicated by the angle formed by joining the a and d triradii to the axis triradius. The more distal the triradius, the greater will be the angle. Normal: less than 57 degrees.

Clearly the more acute this angle, the more proximal will be the triradius; the more obtuse the angle, the higher or more distally will it be found. Angles greater than 56 degrees denote a high triradius.

The position of the triradius, however it be measured, is of value as a physical sign of certain disorders, principally those concerned with chromosome anomalies. While some 3 per cent of normal people may have high or distal triradii, such a position is seven times more likely to be found, let us say, in mongolism than in normal persons. In another chromosome anomaly, trisomy of a D group chromosome (13, 14 or 15) the triradius is likely to be in a very distal situation; similarly the atd angle is very high in the disorder associated with trisomy of chromosome 18.

The rubella-in-utero syndrome shows distal displacement of the axis triradius, and high atd angles tend to be associated with congenital heart disease, more especially with ventricular septal defect and patent ductus arteriosus.

Where the axis triradius is in a distal position true patterns, loops and whorls, are more likely to be found in the ulnar side of the palm, the hypothenar eminence. Thus such hypothenar patterns, as opposed to mere open-fields, are more likely to be found in the chromosome anomalies.

If the ridges that meet at the triradii are traced along their length as "radiants" it will be seen that the long radiant of the a triradius passes away to the hypothenar eminence and the ulnar side of the palm. The long radiant of triradius b passes to the cleft between the ring finger and the little finger, digits IV and V. In so doing it encloses yet another loop formed by the long radiant of the c triradius. In this region, at the base

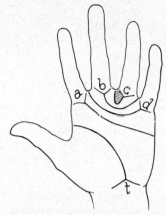

Fig. 32. Third Interdigital Cleft Area. There may or may not be a true pattern in this region.

of the third interdigital cleft there may, or there may not be, a true pattern. True patterns are just a little more likely to occur in mongols than in normal people (Fig. 32).

It has become clear in the last few years that digital and palmar patterns can contribute to clinical diagnosis of chromosomal, and perhaps other, diseases. Dr Irene Uchida of Winnipeg, one of the leading proponents of dermatoglyphic analysis had said: "We have come a long way since the days when we used to receive warm invitations from palmists to join their chiromantic societies!" But we can go a little further yet—by looking at the feet.

The Soles

Up to the present time little attempt has been made to study the patterns on the toes with the same degree of intensity as has been devoted to digital patterns. It is stated that in the condition of trisomy of chromosome 18 arches are found, as on the fingers, with a much increased frequency. It has also been noted that loops open to the fibular or lateral side of the toes are more common among mongols than among controls. Whorls occur much more frequently on the second, third and fourth toes of normal persons than on the toes of mongols whereas whorls are slightly more common on the first toe of mongols than of controls. Despite these well-authenticated differences the toe patterns in our present state of knowledge are less valuable than digital patterns as an aid to diagnosis.

The patterns formed by the ridges on the ball of the foot over the head of the first metatarsal—the hallucal patterns—have been quite extensively studied. Tables have been compiled of the frequencies of whorls, loops large and small, arches open to one side or the other side of the foot, open fields, and other patterns. The size of patterns as measured by ridge counts have also been assessed in relation to chromosome disorders.

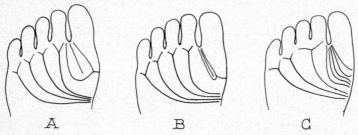

A   B   C

Fig. 33. The Hallucal Area. A shows a large distal loop, B a small distal loop and C a tibial arch. This latter pattern is so uncommon in normals and so frequent in mongols that, of itself, it is of diagnostic value. (*Norma Ford Walker, Pediat. Clin. N. Amer. May 1958, W. B. Saunders Co, Philadelphia*)

The most common normal pattern is the large loop opening distally (41 per cent) (Fig. 33A). Next most common is the whorl (33 per cent). The difference in frequencies between left and right feet is insignificant. Small loops, those with ridge counts below 20 (Fig. 33B) are much less common in normal (10 per cent) than in mongols where they are found with a frequency of 34 per cent. Only 0·9 per cent of mongols have hallucal whorls. Contrast this with the incidence in normals. One can say that an hallucal whorl gives a strong probability against mongolism whereas a small distal loop gives a probability in favour of that diagnosis.

Perhaps the most characteristic pattern of all is the hallucal tibial arch (Fig. 33C). This pattern is extremely rare (0·3 per cent for either foot) in normal persons and yet is the commonest of all patterns found in mongols (47 per cent for either foot). A tibial arch of itself is strongly against the likelihood of normality and greatly in favour of mongolism.

In the other chromosome anomalies unusual patterns may be found.

In cases of the disorder due to trisomy of chromosome 18 an open field on the hallux is common while it is quite rare in normals. In trisomy of one of the D group chromosomes (13, 14 or 15), a fibular arch or a tibial loop may be found, whereas they are uncommon in normals (1·5 per cent and 10 per cent respectively). In the sex chromosome monosomy, X0, very large patterns are found. There are most usually very large whorls or distal loops. One can see, I think, that analyses of dermatoglyphics can help us to a diagnosis. Indeed, using the sixteen areas that we have discussed (neglecting the toe patterns) we can deduce in the case of Down's syndrome such a sure index of probability or unlikelihood that one can make an almost certain diagnosis by mail—by consideration of the dermatoglyphic features of the patient.

Crease Patterns

The major flexion crease patterns of the palms and fingers, which rather surprisingly develop quite early in the foetus and before the ridge

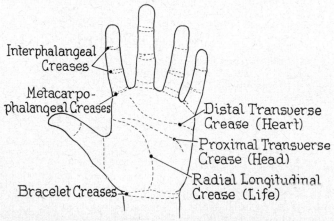

Interphalangeal Creases

Metacarpo-phalangeal Creases

Distal Transverse Crease (Heart)

Proximal Transverse Crease (Head)

Radial Longitudinal Crease (Life)

Bracelet Creases

Fig. 34. Palmar and Digital Skin Creases. These are the lines used by fortune-tellers. While there may be some variation, the distribution is fairly constant. A single interphalangeal crease is suggestive of a chromosome anomaly.

patterns, are fairly constant in their general arrangement though they may differ from one individual to another in points of detail. Some of these creases and their variations are used by palmists in their alleged prognostications as to the future of their possessors. The clinician perhaps is on surer grounds.

Both disciplines recognize the distal wrist crease or "bracelet crease", the most distal crease across the palm (the "line of the heart"), the proximal transverse crease (the "line of the head") and the long line that curves around the thenar eminence: the radial longitudinal crease

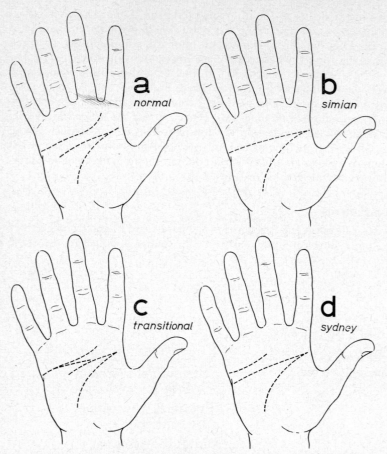

Fig. 35. The Transverse Palmar Crease. Hands a and c are normal. Hand b shows the typical transverse crease or simian crease. It is found in about four per cent of normal persons but is found in about fifty per cent of mongols and certain other chromosome disorders. The sydney line, d, can be regarded as a variant of b and has the same significance.

or "life line". We also recognize the finger flexion creases: the metacarpophalangeal and interphalangeal crease lines (Fig. 34).

In normal persons it is not usual for the distal and proximal transverse creases to be in continuity forming a single crease across the palm. Some 3–4 per cent only of normal persons have such a "Simian crease" or "four finger crease" (Fig. 35b) across their palms. On the other hand 50 per cent of mongols have such a crease on one or other of their hands. Likewise 50 per cent of patients with 18 trisomy have such a crease. Their incidence is much increased in trisomy of a D group chromosome. Such creases are also found in conditions of chromosome deletion: in the X0 monosomy and in the "Cri-du-Chat" syndrome of loss of part of chromosome 5.

Sometimes difficulty can arise in interpreting a palmar crease line, for there are transitional forms (Fig. 35c). Such a crease, while continuous across the palm does not count as a Simian crease. Rather recently a new term has appeared in the chiromantic medical literature: the "Sydney (Australia) line" (Fig. 35d). This crease seems to have roughly the same significance as the transverse palmar or Simian crease. It is rarely seen in normals, but may be seen in cases of mongolism or other chromosome anomaly.

It is exceptional, indeed almost unknown, for a normal person to have but a single digital interphalangeal crease, yet such is found, and not rarely, in the chromosome disorders. Some 20 per cent of mongols have but a single crease on one or other of both of their fifth digits. Perhaps one half of patients trisomic for 18 show such a single crease. The X0 state also quite often shows such a single digital crease.

What can one say in summary of dermatoglyphics as a guide to screening for the chromosome disorders? Perhaps one can say this; consider carefully the possibility of chromosome anomaly in a mentally retarded patient if the following be present: abnormal creases in the palms or a single digit crease, more than six digital arches in a male or more than eight in a female; radial loops on digits IV or V; a tibial arch over a metatarsal head.

Chapter VI
The Incidence of Chromosome Anomalies

The Foetus

Since we have discussed so far only minutiae of cell anatomy and function and tiny details of departure from normal body form the reader may legitimately be wondering if the whole subject of the chromosome disorders might be much ado about nothing: a storm brewed in a teacup. I hope that, by the end of this chapter, he will realize that the chromosome disorders are among the commonest to afflict mankind, and that he will see how very dangerous indeed they are to man.

It is not easy to establish a true incidence. It depends so much on who looks at what sample, where, when and how. There is no such thing as an unselected sample. After all, newborn babies, if chosen as a sample, are selected in that they have been born; that they have lived so long. Having made this admission, we will look at samples of various kinds. Let us start with the foetus, for he after all is of mankind. Unfortunately as yet only the aborted foetus can ethically routinely be examined though special circumstances now justify a chromosome study of selected very young human beings, even in the uterus.

The author's former colleague, David Carr has studied 227 spontaneously aborted foetuses. Fifty-two showed abnormalities of karyotype. Very nearly one quarter. Surely a staggering proportion. Surely an even more staggering number when one remembers that 15 per cent of pregnancies end in miscarriage. Can we say, then, that 4 per cent of mankind, and maybe a good deal more than that if one considers also conceptuses rejected without overt miscarriage, dies early in life of chromosome disorder. I think we can.

What did Carr find? He found, of the 52, that 12 were sex chromosome monosomy XO, 11 were triploid foetuses with three of a kind of each chromosome, nine showed three of a kind of a group E chromosome (they were E trisomies) and there were six each of trisomies of a G group or a D group chromosome. In addition there were two C group trisomics (unidentifiable as to actual chromosome), two tetraploids (four of a kind of all chromosomes) and one each of trisomy number 3, trisomy of a B group member, trisomy of an F chromosome and one trisomic for both a G and an E chromosome. What an amazing collection indeed to find in 227 spontaneously miscarried products of conception!

This probably is an underestimation of total foetal loss due to chromosome anomaly, for Carr also noted that the mean foetal age of the abortions with chromosome anomaly was 86 days whereas the mean age of those abortions without chromosome disorder was 106 days. This suggests that among abortions too young to be recognized as such the incidence of chromosome disorder might well be greater than 25 per cent.

Several similar studies have been made by others. While the incidence of foetal chromosome anomaly, rather curiously, ranged from 8 per cent to 45 per cent, the mean for the pooled data was the same as in Carr's study: 22 per cent.

What does this mean in practical terms? It means this, if nothing else: one can console a patient who has lost a pregnancy as a miscarriage that nature maybe knows best; that, had the pregnancy gone to term, she could have had a severely abnormal baby. The best of the foetuses listed above is the XO monosomy, and even they, if they live, are destined to be sterile. As Carr has said: "We should be thankful that the human uterus can, by some unknown mechanism, prevent the incidence of physical and mental defects reaching astronomical proportion." Amen, to that.

There is a new facet to this matter of chromosome anomaly in the aborted foetus: the "Pill". Oral hormonal contraception is with us to stay, at least until something better comes to hand. Carr has studied its effect on the incidence of chromosome anomaly in the aborted foetuses of mothers who became pregnant within six months of ceasing to take the "pill". Up to November 1968, 29 such abortions have been studied. Ten only were normal. Nineteen of these 29 had a chromosome anomaly. What were they? Twelve were polyploids (an increase in all chromosomes by a multiple of 23); seven triploid for all chromosomes, three tetraploid and two mosaics of the hexaploid (six of all kinds) state. At first sight this looks bad. Fortunately it is not. It is true that the conception after the "pill" is more likely to be miscarried as a polyploid embryo, but since, for practical purposes, no polyploid foetus even reaches term, there is no increased risk (so far as is yet known) of deformed babies as the result of use of the "pill". It is true that in Carr's post-pill abortions there were three XO monosomics and four trisomics, but these numbers are no greater than might be found where the mother had never taken oral contraceptives. So far as present knowledge goes, oral contraceptives do not increase the risk of deformed children; only the risk of foetal loss.

The Newborn: Sex Chromosome Anomalies

Until quite recently we have had only partial knowledge of the incidence of chromosome anomaly in the newborn. One must remember that a full study of a karyotype from a cell culture is a tedious, exacting, and expensive business. Although, through mass production, the cost can be reduced, it is estimated that, in this centre at any rate, a full chromosome analysis costs, in manpower and materials, about $50. This is one reason why full karyotype analyses are rarely applied to large numbers.

Our partial knowledge was gained from an enormous study of the sex

chromatin patterns of buccal mucosal smears of newborns with karyotype analysis of those showing abnormal numbers of Barr bodies.
MacLean and his colleagues in Edinburgh, Scotland, in 1964 published
a report of 10,000 female newborns, and 10,725 males. These figures, not
surprisingly, have not been exceeded since.

Of the 10,000 phenotypic females three were found to be XO and had
detectable abnormalities: webbing of the neck skin or peripheral lym-
phatic oedema. One was judged to be a mosaic with partial deletion of
X in one stem line, and complete absence in the other line: XO/Xx. No
less than 12 in 10,000 were "triple-X", XXX. This, in McLean's study
of liveborn newborns, was by far the most common sex chromosome
anomaly at birth in females. That the XXX constitution was not found
by Carr in his aborted foetuses testifies to the harmless nature of the
X-trisomy. The infrequent finding of the XO constitution in liveborn
females, in contrast with its frequency in Carr's miscarriages, indicates
the lethality of the XO monosomy. Perhaps one out of 40 only of XO
conceptions lives to be born at term.

From MacLean's study of female newborns we can say that in
Scotland, and in the population studied by him, the XO constitution
occurs with a frequency of about one in 2500 births; the XXX in one in
850 births.

Of the 10,725 males, 21 were found to be chromatin positive, indicating that two X chromosomes were present. Investigation of the karyotype indicated that 12 were XXY, one XXYY, three XY/XXY mosaics
and two probably XY/XXY mosaics. In three no karyotype was done,
but they were presumed to have the constitution XXY. None of these
babies, on examination at birth, showed detectable clinical abnormality.
Of the 21 abnormal findings, then, in 10,725 male newborns, 15 were
judged to be XXY, five XY/XXY mosaics and one XXYY; an incidence
altogether of about one in 500 newborn males.

This is not the only big study of sex chromatin in the newborn. In
Denver, Colorado, 15,000 routine buccal smears have been made. The
overall incidence of discrepancy between the expected sex chromatin
and that which was found was 0·17 per cent or about one in 600 babies,
males and females together. In Denver there was an oddity that is as
intriguing as it is difficult to explain. The study was conducted in two
hospitals. Hospital A served a population of higher social and economic
status than Hospital B. The number of babies studied from each hospital was equal. Although the study ran in both institutions from 1964
through (and including) 1967, all aberrations in hospital A were in the
period 1966–67; all aberrations in hospital B were in 1964–65 with
clustering in the months of April and October. In hospital B, no aberrations were discovered in the last 4,800 births whereas in that number
eight might have been found. The authors conclude that their study
indicates "an extremely high degree of probability that the two hospital

populations were exposed in significantly different ways to causes of sex chromosome aberration".

But this is not the only oddity or discrepancy between the expected and the facts. A buccal mucosal study of 2058 males and 1832 female newborns in Bombay, India might, arguing from the data of MacLean in Scotland, have been expected to reveal five chromatin body aberrations. None, in fact, was found. Intruiging, isn't it?

The Newborn: Autosomes and Y Chromosome

Since the Y chromosome and the autosomes cannot be seen in the interphase or resting cell, a study of sex chromatin bodies, the Barr bodies, tells us nothing of autosomal or Y chromosome discrepancies. To learn about these, costly and time-consuming tissue culture methods must be applied.

The largest study of the karyotype of normal newborns has been done in this centre by my colleague Fred Sergovich. He has examined lymphocytic cultures from either the cord blood or capillary blood of 2159 consecutive newborns in one hospital where rich and poor alike are delivered in one obstetrical unit. Cultures grew from 1066 male newborns and from 1015 females. Ten abnormalities were found. They are as follows: phenotypic male babies with the XYY complement, four; XXY, one; trisomy of chromosome 21 with clinical mongolism, two female babies; deletion of part of a B group chromosome with clinical cat-cry syndrome, one; balanced D/D translocation with normal phenotype (see Chapter IV, section on Translocation), one case with mother also a balanced D/D Translocation carrier; unbalanced D/D translocation with D trisomy (see also Translocation, chapter IV), clinical malformations and mother a balanced D/D carrier, one case. No XXX female was found; not surprisingly no XO was revealed.

Unfortunately no other large series is available for comparison. A study of 387 newborns by Turner and Wald showed only one abnormal karyotype, a tetraploid/normal mosaic with normal phenotype.

The best that can be done, failing large neonatal karyotype surveys, is to try to deduce the frequency of abnormality in a population from pooled data of the frequency of occurrence of clinically recognizable abnormalities. Estimates have been made that the incidence of major chromosome abnormality in newborns might be about 0·98 per cent for males and 0·88 per cent for females. The conflict between this estimate and the findings in our series may perhaps best be explained by the fact that our series, though big as such studies go, is too small to permit of statistical validity.

Random Adults

For the reasons of cost and tedium, facts about random adults are quite scanty. A study of chromatin bodies in the buccal smears of 7310 consecutive admissions to an adult hospital revealed seven cases with the constitution XXY and three females who were XXX.

Court Brown has reported a full karyotype study of 438 adults randomly selected from the lists of general practitioners in Edinburgh, Scotland; 207 were men, 231 were women. He divided his findings into three classes: normal, structural abnormalities and re-arrangements, and "variants". He found a balanced D/E reciprocal translocation in a man, a female with a mosaicism of a normal and a D/D translocation stem-line and a man with normal phenotype but with a pericentric inversion (see Chapter IV, Inversion) of the Y chromosome.

In his 438 adult subjects he found 13 "variants". That is to say inherited departures from the usual shape or size of a chromosome without phenotypic abnormality. The most common (and such has been the experience of others) variant was an unusually big Y chromosome: four of the 13 variants. On the basis of this series and of data from other studies he concluded that 0·5 per cent of randomly selected adults have a major chromosome re-arrangement and that 3 per cent of adults show variants.

Perhaps we should here mention that certain circumstances can cause an apparent reduction in the Barr body of sex chromatin. The frequency with which it is found declines with increasing age. It is found in less than the usual number of cells of females around the time of parturition, in those taking antibiotics, those on corticosteroid medication and in those who are severely sick or in a severely stressful situation.

Selected Samples

Although they may be normal phenotypically, certain people or groups of people are at special risk of showing chromosome anomalies on tissue culture of their cells.

Survivors of heavy radiation exposure from the atomic bombings of Hiroshima and Nagasaki have been studied by lymphocytic culture 20 years after the holocausts. From Nagasaki 15 of 43 survivors showed chromosome abnormalities: fragments, ring chromosomes, translocations and inversions. None of a control group showed such abnormalities. Similarly 18 of 51 survivors of Hiroshima, though clinically well, showed similar chromosome damage. Only one of a control series of equal number showed abnormality. Ionizing radiation from other sources than those euphemistically termed "nuclear devices" can lead to chromosome anomalies in the cell cultures of the irradiated.

It has been reported that workers with benzene show chromosome anomalies in the form of excessive numbers of chromosome breaks and recombinations.

Much interest has centred on the effect of the hallucinogen LSD in the last year or two. Some have reported (but others have refuted) that the incidence of chromosome breaks and translocations is four times higher in those taking LSD than in a control population. It has been claimed that the children of LSD users also have an increased incidence of deviant chromosomes. Rebuttal comes from those who contend that the effect of LSD is no more than that of acetylsalicylic acid. In any event, it has been pointed out that those who take LSD may have been abnormal, or from an abnormal environment, before they took the drug. LSD, then, is under unproved suspicion.

So far we have mentioned selection of those who are phenotypically normal. Now just a few words about those who are abnormal. These matters will be discussed again later under appropriate headings.

If one selects the males of childless couples one may find that about 10 per cent have chromosome anomaly. It may be that they are uniformly XXY, but they will be, more probably, mosaics: XO/XY, XY/XXY or such a complicated combination as the mosaic XO/XY/Xx/XxY.

If one selects for low birth weight among newborns at term, it has been experienced in this centre that there is no significant increase in chromosome abnormalities, but if one selects mentally retarded children who were of low birth weight after a full term pregnancy one does find an increase in the incidence abnormalities. Of 150 retarded low birth-weight babies examined here by Dr Chen there were 18 trisomic mongols, and the following occurrences: three XXY, one XO, one XO/XY mosaic, one trisomy of an E group chromosome, a trisomy of a D chromosome, a partial trisomy of B4, a metacentric C group chromosome, a case of cri-du-chat and an inversion of A2. Certainly low birth weight combined with retardation produces a greater yield of chromosome anomalies than retardation alone, for in 150 retardates of normal birth weight, matched with those above for age and sex, Chen found, as with the other group, 18 trisomic mongols but only three, not eleven, others: XXY, XXX and a D/D translocation.

Perhaps the digressions of the later part of this chapter have obscured by now the great significance of chromosomes in relation to disease in man. Let us state, or re-state, the most striking facts. Fifteen per cent of conceptions, at least, end in miscarriage. One quarter of miscarriages are of foetuses with chromosome disorder. Four per cent of human beings (taking a foetus as a human being) die of chromosome disorder before they are even born. About one newborn in every 100, or at the least, 200, has a major chromosome anomaly. Males of an infertile couple have a 10 per cent chance of having a chromosome disorder; where sperms are few or absent the incidence may be double that.

Who now can say that chromosome disorders are unimportant or that cytogenetics deals in trivialities?

Chapter VII
Disorders Due to Autosomal Abnormalities

Mongolism or Down's Syndrome

It seems appropriate, in our descriptions of the clinical abnormalities associated with deviations from the normal morphology or number of the chromosomes, to start with mongolism or, as it is now more fashionable to call it, Down's Syndrome. It shows best the classical features and the variants of a chromosome anomaly. It has been most extensively studied since the first clinical description appeared just over a century ago in the London Hospital Reports.

In 1866 John Langdon Down, while Medical Superintendent of the Earlswood Asylum for Idiots in Surrey, England wrote his now famous paper "Observations on an Ethnic Classification of Idiots". It opens thus:

Those who have given any attention to congenital mental lesions must have been frequently puzzled how to arrange, in any satisfactory way, the different classes of this defect which may come under their observation. Nor will the difficulty be lessened by what has been written on the subject.

One is afraid that this is largely true today although a hundred years have passed. But it is, in fact, a result of Down's own attempt at a new classification that we have come to recognize this well-defined cause of mental retardation.

I have been able to find among the large numbers of idiots and imbeciles that have come under my observation . . . that a considerable portion can be fairly referred to one of the great divisions of the human family other than the class from which they have sprung . . . . Several well-marked examples of the Ethiopian variety have come under my notice, presenting the characteristic malar bones, the prominent eyes, the puffy lips, and the retreating chin . . . . Some arrange themselves around the Malay variety, and present in their soft, black, curly hair, their prominent upper jaws and capacious mouths, types of the family which people the South Sea Islands. Nor have there been wanting the analogues of the people, who with shortened foreheads, prominent cheeks, deep set eyes, and slightly apish nose, originally inhabited the American Continent.

The great Mongolian family has numerous representatives, and it is to this division, I wish, in this paper to call special attention. A very large number of congenital idiots are typical Mongols. So marked is this, that when placed side to side, it is difficult to believe that the specimens compared are not children of the same parents.

He then goes on to describe the typical "mongolian" idiot, mentioning the broad, flat face, the obliquely placed eyes and the heavy epicanthic folds. He draws attention to the thick, fissured lips, the thick rough tongue and the small nose. He describes the skin (perhaps he has erroneously mistaken some hypothyroid cretins for mongols) as having a dirty, yellowish tinge and as being deficient in elasticity. He remarks on their lively sense of the ridiculous, their sense of humour and their aptitude for mimicry. He states, that, while most learn to speak, the speech is thick and indistinct. He hints at their especial liability to winter infections and strongly emphasizes the gains that will result from efforts at training. He gives, indeed, a masterful first description of this syndrome that we have come to know so well.

When he ventures to speculate as to aetiology he goes astray. He makes the good point that "they are always congenital idiots, and never result from accident after uterine life" but he claims that "they are, for the most part, instances of degeneracy arising from tuberculosis in the parents". He appears to regard the condition as a reversion to a primitive mongolian ethnic stock. His son Reginald, himself also a specialist in mental retardation, later repudiated his father's views and wrote: "It would appear that the characteristics which at first sight strikingly suggest mongolian features and build are accidental and superficial being associated, as they are, with other features which are in no way characteristic of that race . . . ."

John Langdon Down considered that "the mongolian type of idiocy occurs in more than 10 per cent of the cases that are presented to me". A report from New York state in 1955 gives the incidence of mongolism among 12,000 retarded children as 9·8 per cent.

Following Down's description one is somewhat surprised how little was added to our knowledge over the next 90 years in spite of an enormous volume of speculation. However, there are some important milestones along the way. In 1876 Fraser and Mitchell pointed out that mongols (for simplicity I will continue to use that term throughout this book) tended to be born at the end of large sibships, while in 1909 Shuttleworth pointed out that this could be the result, perhaps, of maternal age rather than parity.

In the first decade of the 20th century mongolism became divorced from cretinism. Before then the conditions had been confused. It also became accepted that this was not a form of regression to an ancestral ethnic type, but that the resemblance was superficial and fortuitous. It became known that the syndrome could be recognized in Negroes, in Indians and in the Japanese and Chinese peoples.

In 1933, Penrose, who continues to devote his life actively to a study of mongolism, showed that there was indeed a relationship of maternal age to mongolism irrespective of the number of children she had borne. In 1951 he noted that a curve of the incidence of mongolism plotted against maternal age showed two peaks: the one corresponding to the maternal age at which the birth rate is highest (around 25 years), the other corresponding with a maternal age group around 40 years. More-over, he showed that there was a significant lowering of the mean maternal age of the mother at the birth of a mongol child in those families where there was a mongol relative or where the mother had herself previously had a mongol child. There was a hint that there might be two varieties of mongols: those in which the age of the mother was relevant to aetiology and those which were independent of maternal age (Fig. 36).

It had also become known that monozygotic twins were almost in-variably "concordant" for the disease. That it to say, if one of mono-zygotic twins was a mongol the other almost invariably was a mongol also. (We will return to why concordance is not invariable later.) In

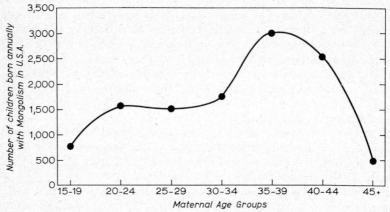

Fig. 36. Number of children with Mongolism born annually in U.S.A. to mothers in the different age groups. (*C. E. Benda, The Child with Mongolism, Grune & Stratton Inc, New York*)

dizygotic twins the concordance was not significantly greater than among non-twin sibs. The disease was clearly of genetic origin, and not due to intra-uterine environmental factors. In addition, it had been noted that in the rare event that a mongol woman had a child the chances for the baby of mongolism or normality were approximately even.

As long age as 1932 de Waadenburg proposed that mongolism might be due to a chromosome abnormality. This was a most prescient but, at that time, unsupported suggestion.

In 1959 Lejeune, Gautier and Turpin in Paris applying the knowledge of the normal array of human chromosomes gained three years prev-iously by Tjio and Levan, showed beyond doubt that there was to be found in the cells of mongols an extra small acrocentric chromosome in group G, by convention number 21. They found trisomy 21 in mongols. They had three of a kind, not a pair. They had 47 chromosomes, not 46.

Soon after this Polani discovered a mongol with 46 chromosomes, and at first sight it would seem that this finding destroyed the concept that mongolism is due to an additional 21 chromosome. But there was a good explanation for this apparent paradox. It could be seen that there was indeed in their case an extra chromosome 21, but that it was joined on to, translocated on to, one of the other chromosomes. The extra chromosome was indeed there, exerting its evil influence in just the same way as if it had been "free".

In 1961 Clarke and her colleagues discovered a child who, while having some features of mongolism, was not typical of the disease. Her I.Q. was normal. They found in this child two cell populations: a stem line trisomic for chromosome 21 and stem line of cells that were quite normal. She was a mixture of two cell stem lines, normal and trisomic. She was a mosaic, a "Mongol Mosaic".

Between 1959 and 1961, then, great advances had been made. The trisomic state for chromosome 21 had been recognized in the great majority of mongols and there had also been recognized the "translocation mongol" and the mongol mosaic. In 1963 Dent announced the discovery of a child who showed an unusually mild degree of mongolian stigmata. In this case, and in other "partial mongols", it was found that only part of a 21 chromosome was present in excess. Dent's child was only trisomic for part of number 21. In 1967 Lejeune and his colleagues described what could be regarded as the counterpart of mongolism, a child with what has been called "anti-mongolism". In this and subsequently described cases, part of a 21 chromosome was missing from the normal pair. There was partial deletion of number 21. To complete the picture of mongolism and its counterparts, Al-Aish and co-workers reported the unique event of a child with 45 chromosomes only, a monosomy of chromosome 21. Truly, if such there can be, the opposite of mongolism.

How many mongols, or potential mongols, are conceived yet fail to be born? This is not easy to answer. In 227 aborted conceptuses Carr found six to be trisomic for a G group chromosome. We cannot say if these were mongol foetuses or not. Chromosome 21, the "Mongol" chromosome and number 22 cannot with certainty be distinguished, but it is at least more than a possibility that mongol foetuses (along with conceptuses with other chromosome anomalies) may be preferentially rejected by miscarriage.

Incidence of Mongolism

One might imagine from all the interest that has been focussed on mongolism in the last 100 years that it is a very common condition. It really is not. About one in every 700 babies born is a mongol. We can put the incidence in proper perspective if we realize that a practitioner handling one delivery a week might see a mongol baby born once every twelve years or so. Congenital heart disease, taking all types together is perhaps four times more common. Cystic fibrosis or mucoviscidosis is perhaps half as common as mongolism. The prevalence of mongolism in, let us say, a school-aged population is a good deal less than one in 700, for about 40 per cent die in the first year, mostly from congenital heart disease which afflicts about one third of mongols.

The condition is recognized in Negroes and is well known among Asiatic races. The incidence is probably much the same as in Caucasians. Some studies have appeared to show a variation in incidence with the season of the year. A study from Australia aroused much interest a couple of years ago, for it claimed to show a relationship between the conception of mongols and an epidemic of infective hepatitis. It was

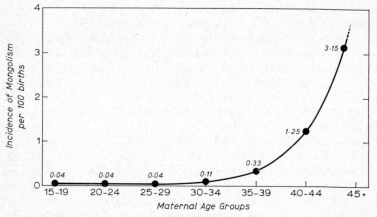

Fig. 37. The incidence of mongolism per one hundred births in different maternal age groups. (*Graph constructed from data by L. S. Penrose, Chap. 13, Human Chromosomal Abnormalities, Charles C. Thomas Publisher, Springfield, Illinois*)

suggested that sub-clinical infective hepatitis predisposed to non-disjunction at meiosis and thus to the occurrence of chromosome trisomy. This exciting observation has not been confirmed but cannot yet be dismissed. There is no increase in the incidence of mongolism in consanguineous marriages.

For several decades it has been known that the incidence of mongolism varies with maternal age, but not with the age of the father. As a woman gets older her chance of having a mongol child rises, irrespective of how many children she previously has had. A young mother of, say, 25 years has a negligible statistical or empiric risk of having a mongol child; perhaps two or three thousand to one against. (Statistical risks, be it noted, do not take into account special cases within a group of young mothers where the risk to the individual may be very high.) The mother of riper years, say aged 40, runs a much greater risk: perhaps 40 or 60 to one against. Fig. 37 shows this increasing risk with age.

There is no doubt that the mother who has had one mongol child, or in whose family there is a mongol relative, has a higher risk of a mongol child—or a second mongol child—than a mother who gives no family history of mongolism. We shall return to this.

Clinical Features

It is not our purpose here to describe exhaustively the clinical features of the disorder. Such descriptions are found in standard texts.

The most striking and distressing feature is the universal mental retardation. The I.Q. varies between 20 and 60 with a mean value around 40. Whether the degree of retardation is determined by differing severity of the disease itself or whether it is largely modified by environment and upbringing it is difficult to say. It seems to me that a mongol born to parents of high intellect, and thus with a better hereditary intellectual potential, is less retarded than one born to dull and backward parents. It has struck me that mongolism seems to cut the potential I.Q. in half. Probably the varying intellectual levels attained are environmentally determined, for it seems that the best can be made of the mongol's potential when he is stimulated, encouraged, kept in his home and loved. However, this may be, even the brightest mongol child will not become a self-supporting citizen.

It is often difficult at first for the parents to accept the diagnosis, for to them the baby shows little evidence of retardation. The mongol is at his best in early infancy, and by comparison with other babies may not appear at this age to be abnormal. As time goes on he falls more and more behind, until by the end of the first year the retardation can scarcely be denied by even the most optimistic parent.

There is one bright side to this sad picture. The mongol child is a happy child, affable, humorous and most affectionate. They are not continually crying, whining, destructive and evil-tempered as are some other retarded children. They are easy to handle in the home, loveable and often much loved.

Their parents are naturally concerned with walking, speech and toilet training. Walking may be delayed to two years or more; but they all walk. Speech development is always slow; but almost all will talk but almost always the voice is thick and gutteral; phrases and words are simple. Toilet training, like walking, takes time but almost all achieve good control.

The appearance is striking (Fig. 38) and yet it is as difficult to say just what makes a child look like a mongol as it is to say, in factual terms, just what makes a pretty girl look pretty. Analysis of individual features does not help too much. It is the whole impression that makes for the diagnosis of mongolism—and that of the pretty girl.

Rather surprisingly there has been no certain portrayal of a mongol in art down through the ages, and this has led to the question; is mongolism a disease of only recent appearance? This is quite unlikely. To the author the idiot in the 16th century picture by Hieronymus Bosch of a quack surgeon removing the "stone of folly" looks like an adult mongol.

Mongols are small. The mean birth weight in a series of mongols in this centre was six pounds, nine ounces (normal, seven pounds, two

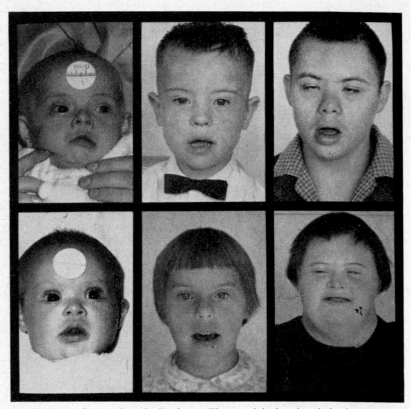

Fig. 38. Mongolism or Down's Syndrome. The top right-hand male is about eighteen years old, the bottom right female is middle-aged. The discs on the foreheads of the babies are for identification in a survey.

ounces). Throughout life they remain of short stature. At least three quarters are under the average height for age. Few adult mongols are over five feet tall. In relation to height they tend to be overweight.

Hypotonia is a striking and constant feature of the young mongol child. They are extremely floppy; their joints may be hyperextended and their limbs placed in grotesque positions. Just recently this hypotonia has become of interest, for it has been claimed that the administration of 5-hydroxytryptophane (a precursor of serotonin) abolishes or much reduces this hypotonia. Time will tell if this observation can be confirmed or if it is of value as a form of therapy.

"Acromicria", an alternative name that has been suggested for this syndrome describes the shortness of limbs especially of the distal bones, that is largely responsible for the short stature. The hands are rather square and the fingers short and stubby. The little finger may be very short and somewhat incurved, though this is not so valuable a sign as some would lead one to suppose. The whole hand is extraordinarily flabby and has a unique soft feel. The feet are short and broad with a

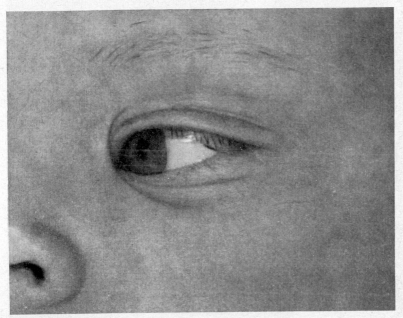

Fig. 39. Epicanthic Fold in Normal Child. This feature is so common in normal infants that its presence in Mongolism is of dubious diagnostic significance.

poorly developed arch. There is often a wide gap between the big toe and the toe next to it.

The head is small and rather square, foreshortened from front to back, brachycephalic. The neck is short and thick. The eyes are set closer together than is normal because of the underdevelopment of the skull. The orbital sockets, as seen in an X-ray are small and oval. The ears are set low in the head, and are of unusual shape: small, rounded or nearly square in childhood, though they may become large and floppy in adult life.

The eyes, in childhood at any rate, are slanted upwards at the outer side. This feature becomes less obvious in later life. Most writings mention an epicanthic fold of skin, a crescentic fold running from the upper lid to the nasal bridge, covering in part the lachrimal caruncle. While this skin fold is present in most young mongols, I do not believe that this sign has any value. It is so common in quite normal infants that its presence in a mongol seems irrelevant (Fig. 39). The iris is more usually

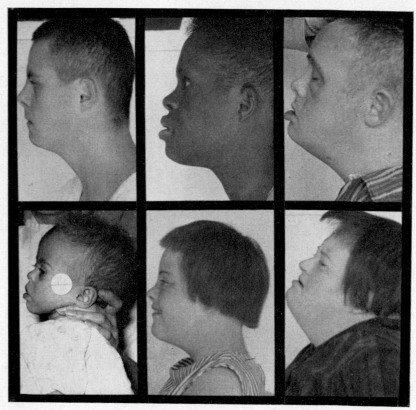

Fig. 40. Six Examples of Mongolism or Down's Syndrome. The slope of the submental region and the tendency to "double chin" is very constant. The male, upper right, and the female, lower right, are middle-aged.

blue or grey than in the population as a whole, and in the blue or grey-eyed mongol small white speckles are often found around the periphery for a variable length of the circumference. These Brushfield spots, though found in nearly one-half of mongols are present sometimes in normal persons; thus they lack diagnostic value. Squints are common, and in later years degenerative opacities of the lens are often found. In later years, also, many mongols have chronic blepharitis.

The nose is often small, and the patient is plagued with persistent obstruction and infection. The mongol child snorts and snuffles his way from one infection to the next. It is possible that the small size of the post-nasal space and airway is responsible. The tongue, too large for the small mouth, often protudes, and perhaps as the result of constant exposure to the air, becomes thickened, fissured and, as it has been called, "scrotal". The lips are thick and fissured, and in older children and in adults the lower lip may become large and hang down. There is often malocclusion of the teeth, but the teeth themselves seem especially resistant to dental caries. The chin recedes somewhat, and the neck below the chin becomes filled in with redundant tissue, giving often a "double chin" (Fig. 40). The trunk is not especially unusual though the nipples are rather flat. In females pubertal breast development is delayed by several years, but in mongol women the breasts often become large with fat and pendulous. Congenital heart disease of various types is common. Perhaps nearly 50 per cent have heart defects of one kind or another. The large cushion septal defect, the atrioventricularis communis, is perhaps the most common. The tetralogy of Fallot with cyanosis is not rare.

Anomalies of the gastrointestinal tract are quite uncommon, but one especially deserves mention: atresia of the duodenum. If a mongol has a neonatal bowel obstruction, one must think that the lesion may be a duodenal atresia. If a newborn is found to have atresia of the duodenum, one must think that the baby might be a mongol.

The male genitalia are often abnormal for there may be permanently undescended testes and a tiny penis. Puberty is often much delayed, and in males testicular degeneration and infertility seem to be the rule. The female genitalia are said to show large cushion-like labia majora and small insignificant labia minora. These features are not too striking. Puberty and menarche are usually much delayed and menstruation when it comes is irregular and the menopause comes early.

The pelvis shows some unusual features (Fig. 41). The iliac wings are wide and flat. They overhang the acetabulum making the "acetabular angle" narrow. The iliac angle also is smaller than normal.

It is a curious fact that acute leukaemia is at least three (some have said 20) times more common in the mongol than in normals. Many of the rather few reported cases of neonatal leukaemia have occurred in mongols. Some have said that the increased incidence of leukaemia is not specific for mongolism and that there is an increased risk in any chromosome disorder. This may or may not be true, but it is a well-established fact that in another variety of leukaemia that affects adults only, chronic myeloid leukaemia, there is a chromosome abnormality in the cells of the peripheral blood. A tiny chromosome fragment, the Philadelphia Chromosome, is all that remains of one small acrocentric believed to be number 21, the chromosome relevant to mongolism. This can scarcely be coincidence.

It is also known that in chronic myeloid leukaemia the alkaline phosphatase activity of the blood leucocytes is reduced. On this evidence it
was suggested that the gene for such enzyme activity might be on the
deleted part of chromosome 21. It was suggested that the gene locus for
cell alkaline phosphatase activity was on the 21 chromosome. It looked
as though this might be the case indeed when it was found that the
levels of alkaline phosphatase were in fact higher in the mongol who, of

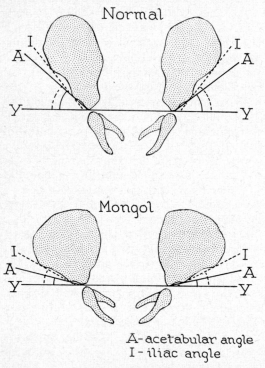

A-acetabular angle
I-iliac angle

Fig. 41. Acetabular and Iliac Angles in Normals and in Mongols. Both angles are
diminished in mongolism. (*J. Caffey and S. Ross*, The Pelvis in Mongolism, Ped.
17 : 642, 1956. *Charles C. Thomas Publisher, Springfield, Illinois*)

course, has the relevant chromosome in excess. Unfortunately this
localization has been refuted by the finding that there is a similar rise of
phosphatase in other chromosome anomalies. The effect is non-
specific. Moreover in the mongol a number of enzymes show a rise in
concentration, including even glucose-6-phosphate dehydrogenase which
is known for certain to be carried on the X chromosome.

Quite recently a strange new observation has been made. In eight of
eight mongols studied (and in only one of eight controls) a tiny oblong
crystalline body could be seen in the cytoplasm of cultured lympho-

cytes. This may be an aggregation of virus particles. It may represent a large protein molecule. We await more news of this with interest.

We must, I'm afraid, admit that we do not know just what the underlying defects may be. We do not know why some unfortunate mothers suffer non-disjunction at meiosis while others of comparable age do not. Although there does seem, as we have mentioned, to be a weak familiality (a slight extra risk of recurrence in a family) of non-disjunction mongolism, we do not know why. If reproductive performance, fertility and miscarriage can be taken as an indication of liability to produce chromosomally abnormal conceptuses, there seems to be no especial risk in mothers of mongols. A study of this matter by my colleague, Professor Carol Buck and by myself showed no impairment of reproductive performance. A detailed comparison of 22 features of body form and measurement of parents and sibs of mongols with closely matched boys, girls, men and women without a mongol in the family showed nothing unusual about the mongol families. But one thing has been noted by several workers. There is an increased incidence of thyroid disease in the mothers of mongols and in her near relatives: hyperthyroidism, hypothyroidism and goitre. Even if there is no overt thyroid disease there is undoubtedly an increased incidence of the occurence of thyroglobulin auto-antibodies in mothers (especially young mothers) of mongols, sibs of mongols, near relatives of mongols and in the mongols themselves. Curious, but perhaps not specific for mongolism. An increased frequency of thyroid auto-antibodies is found also in mothers of XO monosomies.

Even as we do not know why non-disjunction and trisomy comes about, we do not know why trisomy 21 has the effects it does. We can only vaguely say that an imbalance of genetic material must exist, and that that imbalance causes a multiplicity of defects.

The average expectation of life for the mongol is short for many die of heart disease in the first year. Better nursing care and the antibiotics have so reduced the hazards of respiratory infection that the outlook for survival may not be much reduced once the dangerous first year is passed.

Questionable Mongols, Partial Trisomy, Mosaics

Is mongolism an "all or none" condition? Is the patient an undoubted mongol, or not a mongol at all? Are there degrees of mongolism? In general the condition is absolute with perhaps some variation especially in intellect, as the result of hereditary and environmental influences for good or ill. But there are exceptions. There are semi- or partial mongols.

Patrick F. was watched by an experienced paediatrician for three years. Was he, he wondered, or was he not, a mongol? (Fig. 42a.) He was sent to me for an opinion. The more I looked the less certain did I become. For a fleeting moment one would see him as an undoubted mongol; in the next moment that im-

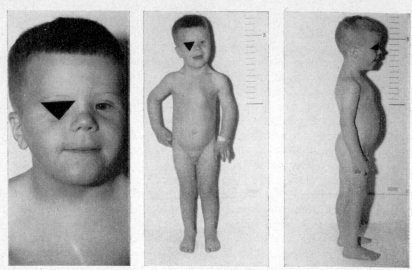

Fig. 42a. Patrick F. Is he, or is he not, a mongol? This question much puzzled his pediatrician, Dr W. Stein of Kitchener, Ontario. Chromosome studies showed that he is a translocation "semi-mongol" with part of an extra 21 chromosome present and translocated to a D group chromosome. (*F. Sergovich, H. Valentine, D. Carr, and H. Soltan, J. Pediat, 65(2) : 197, 1964. C. V. Mosby Company, St Louis, Missouri*)

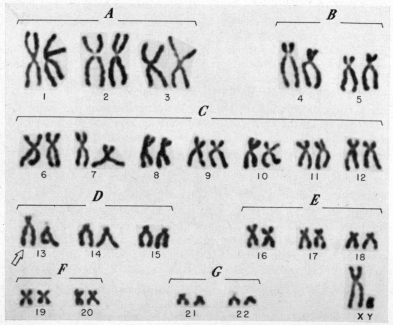

Fig. 42b. Patrick F. Karyotype. Two "free" 21 chromosomes and part of an additional 21 chromosome translocated on to a D group chromosome. A "semi-mongol". (*Preparation by Dr D. H. Carr*)

pression had gone. He was at the borderline level of intelligence and his dermatoglyphic patterns were typical of mongolism. Was he or was he not a mongol? Chromosome analysis showed part, but not the whole of an extra chromosome 21 in the karyotype of his peripheral blood (Fig. 42b). He was a true "semi-mongol".

Stephen C. a retarded boy of seven years of age, had been regarded, by the highly experienced staff of a Hospital School for the Retarded, as a mongol. When presented to this author and his colleagues there was much debate and a division of opinion. Dermatoglyphic patterns were in some respects indicative of mongolism but were not truly diagnostic. A single crease only was found on the fifth digit of one hand. Such a feature is found in 20 per cent of

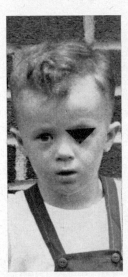 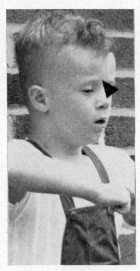 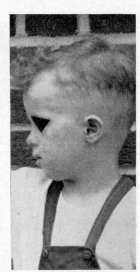

Fig. 43. Stephen C. Is he, or is he not, a mongol? He had been regarded as such by very experienced clinicians. Chromosome studies did not show any visible abnormality. Is he a mongol mosaic? We do not know. (*F. Sergovich, H. Valentine, D. Carr, H. Soltan, J. Pediat, 65(2) : 197, 1964. C. V. Mosby Company, St Louis, Missouri*)

mongols, but is never seen in normals. Was he a mongol (Fig. 43). Analyses of several tissues showed normal numbers and morphology of the chromosomes. Is he a mongol? Is he a mongol mosaic? This we can never know for we cannot be sure that there is not an abnormal stem line of cells somewhere in his body tissues. One can never prove that a person is not a mosaic; one can only sometimes prove that he is one.

We do not know if Stephen is a mongol mosaic, but we do know that mosaicism for a 21 trisomy stem line can result in mongolism that may, presumably depending on the proportions of normal and abnormal cells, be either fully developed mongolism or mongolism of modified degree. (For mechanism of normal/trisomy mosaicism, see Fig. 21B and text).

Irene Uchida in a recent study of 453 mongols found five mongol mosaics.

It seems then that the phenotypic expression of mongolism may be related to gene dosage. Three 21 chromosomes gives a full-blooded mongol. Less than complete trisomy may give modified mongolism, and less than the full trisomic state may come about in two ways. Every cell may contain part of an extra 21 chromosome or "partial trisomy", or there may be mosaicism of normal cells and fully trisomic cells.

There are, then, cases where the diagnosis can be in doubt, but they are extremely rare.

"Anti-Mongolism"

Having said that the expression of mongolism can be dependent on doseage of extra genetic material, it is legitimate to enquire what happens if there is less than the normal amount of material of chromosome 21. Cases have been reported recently.

Lejeune has reported a mosaic monosomic for chromosome 21 in one stem line but with the other stem line normal. Kasahara has reported partial loss of chromosome 21 in every cell.

The features of these extraordinary cases have been something which has been termed the mongol "contre-type" or "anti-mongolism". The ears are large and floppy, not small. The eyes slope downwards at the outer side, the nose is big. Simian palmar creases are not reported. There is muscle hypertonia not hypotonia. There is thrombocytopaenia and this is not a feature of the mongol child. There is a remarkably high incidence of pyloric stenosis, a condition that is said to be unusually uncommon in mongols.

Here the dissimilarity to mongolism seems to end. Like the mongol they tend to have heart deformities, they have, like the mongol, rather receding chins. Unfortunately, in common with the mongol they are mentally retarded.

As mentioned at the beginning of this chapter one child has been described who is uniformly monosomic for chromosome 21. This was a unique discovery for, up to that time, it had been believed that monosomy of an autosome (as opposed to the sex chromosome monosomy XO) was incompatible with any form of existence. No autosome monosomy was found even in Carr's aborted foetuses.

The single child with monosomy 21 (or at least of a G group chromosome thought to be 21) was alive at four and a half years; mentally retarded, with seizures, hemiparesis, small mouth, small low-set ears, and downward-sloping eyes. There was no heart lesion and the dermatoglyphic patterns, apart from wide atd angles were unremarkable. Indeed the whole picture of this 21 monosomic child was rather non-specific.

It seems that chromosome 21 either is somewhat poorly endowed with gene material or that its genes are somewhat unimportant. Of the autosomal trisomics only mongolism is compatible with more than a few months or years of life; monosomy 21 is the only complete autosomal monosomy reported in the living. After this digression, let us return to mongolism.

Dermatoglyphics in Mongolism

As has been mentioned, the dermal ridge patterns on the finger tips, palms and soles of a mongol of any age are different from those of the normal to such a degree that, given good prints, a diagnosis of mongolism can be made with considerable reliability in the absence of the patient himself. The method works thus.

Table 3

	DIGITS, LEFT HAND									
	V		IV		III		II		I	
PATTERN	Mongol	Normal	Mongol	Normal	Mongol	Normal	Mongol	Normal	Mongol	Normal
Whorl	18·3	12·0	32·8	36·9	13·6	17·4	11·9	33·4	22·4	30·8
Ulnar Loop	77·1	85·4	58·7	60·2	83·5	71·4	82·4	36·3	73·0	62·7
Radial Loop	2·9	0·1	5·1	0·9	1·7	2·6	2·3	19·4	0·6	0·8
Arch	1·7	2·6	3·4	3·0	1·1	8·6	3·4	10·9	4·0	5·8

	DIGITS, RIGHT HAND									
	I		II		III		IV		V	
PATTERN	Mongol	Normal	Mongol	Normal	Mongol	Normal	Mongol	Normal	Mongol	Normal
Whorl	25·9	38·6	14·9	35·7	11·3	18·4	31·8	46·6	18·9	14·6
Ulnar Loop	70·6	57·3	82·3	31·1	86·4	70·9	60·2	52·0	75·4	84·0
Radial Loop	0·1	0·8	1·7	20·3	1·1	3·4	5·7	0·3	4·6	0·3
Arch	3·5	3·3	1·1	12·9	1·1	6·3	2·3	1·1	1·1	1·1

Percentage frequencies of digital patterns for each digit of both hands in mongols and normals. (*Norma Ford Walker, Pediat. Clin. N. Amer. May 1958, W. B. Saunders Co, Philadelphia*)

If one takes the first digit, the thumb, of the right hand, tables derived from the study of many normal persons will tell us that whorls, ulnar loops, radial loops, and arches will be found in respective percentages thus: 38·6, 57·3, 0·8, 3·3 (Table 3). In mongols the respective frequencies are different: 25·9 per cent, 70·6 per cent, 0·1 per cent, 3·5 per cent. If an ulnar loop, then, is found on the first digit, the probability that our patient is a mongol is as 70·6 is to 57·3; a probability of 1·23 to 1. If we now take the second digit of the right hand, the index finger, we have normal ratios thus: whorls 35·7 per cent, ulnar loops 31·1 per cent, radial loops 20·3 per cent and arches 12·9 per cent. In mongols the ratios are respectively 14·9 per cent 82·3 per cent, 1·7 per cent, and 1·1

Table 4

PATTERN	DIGITS, LEFT HAND				
	V	IV	III	II	I
Whorl	1·53	0·89	0·78	0·36	0·73
Ulnar Loop	0·90	0·97	1·17	2·27	1·16
Radial Loop	29·00	5·67	0·65	0·12	0·75
Arch	0·65	1·70	0·13	0·31	0·69

PATTERN	DIGITS, RIGHT HAND				
	I	II	III	IV	V
Whorl	0·67	0·43	0·58	0·68	1·29
Ulnar Loop	1·23	2·65	1·22	1·16	0·90
Radial Loop	0·13	0·08	0·32	19·00	15·33
Arch	1·06	0·09	0·17	2·09	1·10

Ratios of percentage frequencies of digital patterns: frequency in mongols divided by frequency in normals. (*Norma Ford Walker, Pediat. Clin. N. Amer. May 1958, W. B. Saunders Co, Philadelphia*)

per cent. It is easy to see that an arch on the second digit gives a high probability for normality, while an ulnar loop gives a probability for mongolism of 82·3 to 31·1, or 2·65 to 1.

In this way we can examine all ten digits and determine for each digit the probability or otherwise for mongolism, depending on the pattern found (Table 4). Making the assumption (and some have questioned this) that the patterns on each finger are independently derived, one can determine a total index of probability of mongolism or normality by the multiplication of the individual probabilities. A "digital index" can be deduced.

To make things easy for us, those who have devised such tables have, of the kindness of their heart, converted the probability values to logarithms (Table 5). To multiply a series of numbers together is tedious. To add them is easy. Expressed as logarithms it comes to the same thing. To get our index we simply add together the logarithms of the probabilities given in Table 5.

If we now look at Fig. 44 we can see how likely, or unlikely, it may be that our patient is a mongol. If the logarithmic digital index is, let us

Table 5

PATTERN	DIGITS, LEFT HAND				
	V	IV	III	II	I
Whorl	+ 0·18	− 0·05	− 0·11	− 0·44	− 0·14
Ulnar Loop	− 0·05	− 0·01	+ 0·07	+ 0·36	+ 0·06
Radial Loop	+ 1·46	+ 0·75	− 0·19	− 0·92	− 0·12
Arch	− 0·19	+ 0·23	− 0·89	− 0·51	− 0·16

PATTERN	DIGITS, RIGHT HAND				
	I	II	III	IV	V
Whorl	− 0·17	− 0·38	− 0·24	− 0·17	+ 0·11
Ulnar Loop	+ 0·09	+ 0·42	+ 0·09	+ 0·06	− 0·05
Radial Loop	− 0·89	− 1·10	− 0·49	+ 1·28	+ 1·19
Arch	+ 0·03	− 1·05	− 0·77	+ 0·32	+ 0·04

Logarithms of ratios shown in Table 4. (*Norma Ford Walker, Pediat. Clin. N. Amer. May 1958, W. B. Saunders Co, Philadelphia*)

say, minus 1·8, it is most unlikely that our patient is a mongol. Very few mongols have such a value. It is not impossible; only most unlikely. On the other hand a value of, shall we say, plus 1·02 is not of much help. Both mongols and normals may have such a value. But we can do better with more data.

Table 6 gives probabilities, or otherwise, for mongolism based on the position of the axis triradius expressed as a percentage of the palm length (Fig. 30). We can see that a high triradius (over 40 per cent, t″) makes mongolism probable in a ratio of roughly eight to one and six

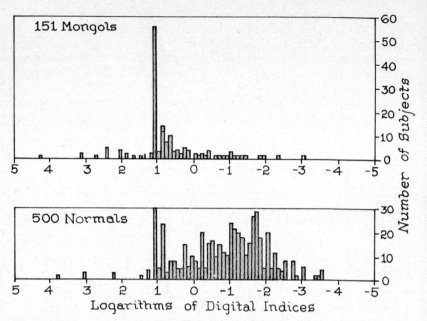

Fig. 44. Histogram of summation of logarithms of the ten digital ratios in mongols and in normals. This figure shows the distribution of these logarithm summations: the "Digital Indices". (*Norma Ford Walker, Pediat. Clin. N. Amer. May 1958, W. B. Saunders Co, Philadelphia*)

to one, on left hands and right hands respectively. Table 7 gives logarithmic values to be added to our digital index derived above.

The presence of a true pattern in the third interdigital cleft—or its absence—gives a further loading for, or against, the possibility of mongolism. The probability in favour of mongolism, where a true pattern is present, is not great; but every little helps. Table 8 gives the percentage

Table 6

Height of Axis Triradius: Position as Percentage of Palm Length	Percentage Frequencies				Ratios of Percentage Frequencies	
	Left Palm		Right Palm		Left	Right
	Mongol	Normal	Mongol	Normal		
Low, under 40%	14·2	89·8	15·6	86·7	0·2	0·2
High, 40% and over	85·8	10·2	84·4	13·3	8·4	6·3

Percentage frequencies of high and low axis triradii for each palm in mongols and in normals. Also the ratios of those frequencies: mongol frequency divided by normal frequency. (*Norma Ford Walker, Pediat. Clin. N. Amer. May 1958, W. B. Saunders Co, Philadelphia*)

Table 7

Height of Axis Triradius	Left	Right
Low, under 40%	– 0·70	– 0·70
High, 40% and over	+ 0·92	+ 0·89

Logarithms of ratios shown in Table 6. (*Norma Ford Walker, Pediat. Clin. N. Amer. May 1958, W. B. Saunders Co, Philadelphia*)

ratios, and Table 9 their logarithms; again to be added to our growing "total index". Now let us look at the hallucal area of the sole, and at the ratios of the patterns in mongols and in controls. Table 10 gives the percentage ratios, Table 11 their logarithmic values. Again this logarithmic value, determined by observation of the pattern, is added to the

Table 8

Configurations, True Pattern or no True Pattern	Percentage Frequencies				Ratios of Percentage Frequencies	
	Left Space		Right Space		Left	Right
	Mongol	Normal	Mongol	Normal		
True Loop or Whorl	54·0	31·3	85·4	55·5	1·7	1·5
Open field, Incomplete Loops	46·0	68·7	14·6	44·5	0·7	0·3

Percentage frequencies of true patterns in the third interdigital space, and ratios of those frequencies: mongol frequency divided by normal frequency. (*Norma Ford Walker, Pediat. Clin. N. Amer. May 1958, W. B. Saunders Co, Philadelphia*)

Table 9

Configurations	Left	Right
True Pattern	+ 0·23	+ 0·18
No True Pattern	– 0·15	– 0·52

Logarithms of ratios shown in Table 8. (*Norma Ford Walker, Pediat. Clin. N. Amer. May 1958, W. B. Saunders Co, Philadelphia*)

value derived from the data from the hand. Now 16 areas have been assessed, and 16 ratios of probability derived. The "total index" is the product of those 16 observations; or the sum of their logarithmic values.

If we now look at histograms (Fig. 45), based on the logarithmic values of those 16 variables, we can get much help towards a diagnosis. Suppose our calculated value, the sum of the 16 logarithmic components, is minus 6·3, we can see that this individual is normal, almost for sure. A value of plus 6·3 makes our patient a mongol almost for certain. If a patient possesses "the most mongol" feature of each of the 16 variables, he could amass a total index of log. plus 10·3. Expressed in actual probabilities he would have, in theory at any rate, a two

Table 10

Pattern on Hallucal area: "Ball" of Foot	Percentage Frequencies				Ratios	
	Left Hallux		Right Hallux		Left	Right
	Mongol	Normal	Mongol	Normal		
Arch,tibial	46·6	0·3	47·4	0·3	155·3	158·0
Loop distal, small	33·8	10·0	31·2	13·3	3·4	2·3
Loop distal, large	12·7	41·0	13·6	42·0	0·3	0·3
Loop distal, incomplete	3·4	0·1*	3·4	0·1*	34·0	34·0
Loop, tibial	2·6	10·0	0·9	9·7	0·2	0·1
Whorl	0·9	33·7	2·6	29·7	0·03	0·1
Tented arch	0·1*	0·3	0·9	0·1*	0·3	9·0
Arch, fibular	0·1*	1·4	0·1*	1·7	0·1	0·1
Loop, fibular	0·1*	0·9	0·1*	1·0	0·1	0·1
Open field	0·1*	3·0	0·1*	2·7	0·03	0·04

Percentage frequencies of hallucal patterns in mongols and in normals. Also ratios of those frequencies: mongol frequency divided by normal frequency. A "large" distal loop has a ridge count of 21 or more. * indicates an assigned value since the observed frequency was zero. (*Norma Ford Walker. Pediat. Clin. N. Amer. May 1958, W. B. Saunders Co, Philadelphia*)

thousand million to one chance in favour of being a mongol. I do not think we can interpret the data in the tables thus literally. One cannot say, for example, that a value of plus log. 6·3 means that the patient has truly a chance of two million to one favour of mongolism; or with a value of log. minus 6·3, a two million to one chance against that diagnosis. One can only look at the histogram (Fig. 45) and see in what zone the index of our patient is to be found. If the value falls within the grey area of the histogram, the likelihood of mongolism—or otherwise—is very high indeed. There is remarkably little overlap. Dr Norma Ford

Walker, from whose writings these tables have been purloined, claimed in 1958: "a new method is outlined by which a purely objective diagnosis of mongolism can be made". Experience has shown this claim to be justified.

Although this knowledge of the tiny dermal ridge patterns is of quite recent date, the transverse palmar crease, the "simian crease", or the "four-finger crease" have been of interest to clinicians for some time. In a recent series of 184 mongols studied by Dr Irene Uchida, and my colleague Dr Hubert Soltan, a transverse crease was found on at least

Table 11

Hallucal Patterns	Left	Right
Arch,tibial	+2·19	+2·20
Loop distal,small	+0·53	+0·36
Loop distal,large	−0·52	−0·52
Loop distal,incomplete	+1·53	+1·53
Loop,tibial	−0·70	−1·00
Whorl	−1·52	−1·00
Tented arch	−0·52	+0·95
Arch,fibular	−1·00	−1·00
Loop,fibular	−1·00	−1·00
Open field	−1·52	−1·40

Logarithms of ratios shown in Table 10. (*Norma Ford Walker, Pediat. Clin. N. Amer. May 1958, W. B. Saunders Co, Philadelphia*)

one hand in 74 patients (40 per cent), as compared with 28 (4 per cent) on the hands of 685 non-mongol persons. A transverse palmar crease, then, gives a probability of 10 to 1 in favour of mongolism. It is not diagnostic. It is suggestive only. On one occasion, of nine of my medical students, three had a transverse palmar crease. This was admittedly a long coincidence.

A single crease on the fifth, or any other, digit is much more suggestive of mongolism or some other chromosome anomaly. It is extremely rarely, if ever, found in normal persons. In a mongol it is found on one hand or the other in 20 per cent of patients. This is an important sign.

If we have dealt at what seems undue length on dermal ridge patterns,

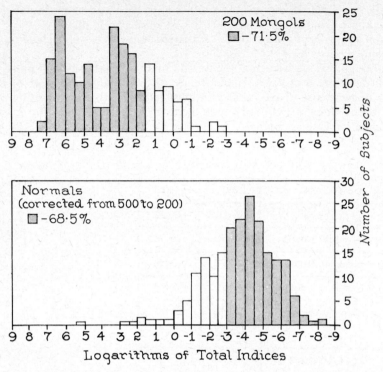

Fig. 45. Histogram of summation of logarithms of the sixteen dermal areas, mongols and normals. This figure shows the distribution of the "Total Index". (*Norma Ford Walker, Pediat. Clin. N. Amer. May 1958, W. B. Saunders Co, Philadelphia*)

it is because I wish to illustrate a method of diagnosis which is not as yet to be found in standard tests. Details are given in the expectation that readers might be interested to apply these methods to any patient under their care. They will be found to work.

Cytogenetic Mechanisms in Mongolism

Chromosomally speaking there are several varieties of mongol. There is the "regular" trisomy 21 mongol. There is the "de novo" translocation mongol, the hereditary translocation mongol and, as a very rare event, the mongol due to formation of an isochromosome of both long arms of number 21. The first is by far the most common. There are even, as we have seen, varying degrees of mongolism, though partial mongols are really quite uncommon.

The frequency with which the various types are found depends on the method of selection of the cases studied. If the mongol children of older mothers only were to be studied almost all would be found to be of the regular trisomic variety for it is this type that is related to maternal age. The older the mother, the more likely is it that she will bear a mongol child, and the more likely is it that this will be caused by non-disjunction at meiosis. If, on the other hand, the cases selected for study are predominantly the mongol children of young mothers, a significant proportion of examples of mongolism of non-trisomic type will be found. Again, if the sample is selected from those families where there is a sib or relative with mongolism a significant number of cases will be found where the mechanism is something other than primary non-disjunction; but, even so, the non-disjunction trisomic mongols will greatly outnumber all other varieties together.

In the largest series studied, the 453 mongols of Irene Uchida of Winnipeg, 13 were mongols with translocation; of those nine were "de novo" (to be discussed later) and four were by inheritance from a balanced translocation carrier (see Chapter IV, gametogenesis in balanced translocation). There were five trisomy/normal mosaics, one mongol by isochromosome formation (Fig. 16A, B) and one with a double trisomy: trisomy 21 and XXY. Let us say that 96 per cent of mongols are of trisomic type.

The "Regular" Mongol, Trisomy 21

As we have seen in an earlier chapter (Figs. 10a, b) the gametes, sperm and ova are formed by reduction division at meiosis. It will be recalled that this takes place in two stages, the first and second meiotic divisions. It can come about at either of these divisions (probably most usually the first) that there is incorrect segregation or migration of the chromosomes into the daughter cells of that division. Non-disjunction may occur as shown in Fig. 18A, B. One gamete will have a chromosome too many, both of the pair; the other will have one too few, with no representative of the non-disjuncting pair.

Fertilization of these gametes must result in abnormal zygotes. The one will have three representatives of the relevant pair, the other but one. There will be trisomic and monosomic zygotes. If number 21 is the relevant pair the trisomic zygote is destined to be a mongol (Fig. 46). The monosomic zygote will, with the unique exception mentioned a little earlier, die and be reabsorbed; not even noted as a miscarriage.

What causes such non-disjunction and what causes the relation to maternal age? We just don't know. It is too facile to speak of this as chance mishap. Mishaps must have a cause. We can, it is true, relate an increased risk of non-disjunction to maternal age by postulating that the long, long prophase of meiosis, the state of suspended animation of the ovum before the first meiotic division at ovulation, so alters segregation of the chromosomes that non-disjunction is more likely to occur. This may be the truth, but there are other possibilities. Maybe with advancing years (and sometimes in young mothers for other and unknown reasons) there is delay in fertilization of the ovum because passage into the Fallopian tube is slowed. Maybe it is an ovum that has grown overly old after ovulation that suffers non-disjunction when the second meiotic division is started by the stimulus of entry of a sperm. Delayed fertilization in rabbits leads to abnormal segregation of chromosomes and to abnormal zygotes.

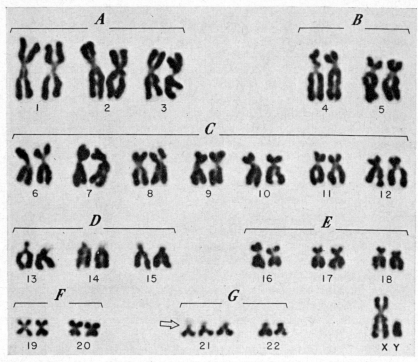

Fig. 46. Karyotype of Trisomic Mongol showing the three chromosomes in one of the sets of group G chromosomes. By convention the chromosome involved in mongolism is called number 21 although it is indistinguishable from number 22. The patient is a male, XY. (*Preparation kindly supplied by Dr F. Sergovich*)

What about the father? It is of course quite possible that non-disjunction occurs at spermatogenesis, but as we have said before, sperms are freshly made in constantly replenished supply. There is no long prophase of meiosis and non-disjunction is, for that reason perhaps, less likely. At least one sees no varying frequency of mongolism with varying paternal age. Maybe non-disjunction does occur at spermatogenesis and that some sperms do contain an extra chromosome. Maybe such sperms, like racehorses carrying too much weight, lag far behind the field in the race for the receptive ovum. Maybe there is such "gamete selection".

"De Novo Translocation" Mongols

The next genetic mechanism that we must consider is the "de novo translocation", for while relatively rare it causes the next most common variety after the trisomic mongol. In Uchida's 453 mongols, nine were mongols with "de novo" translocation; that is to say an extra chromosome attached to another without abnormality of the chromosome complement of the parents.

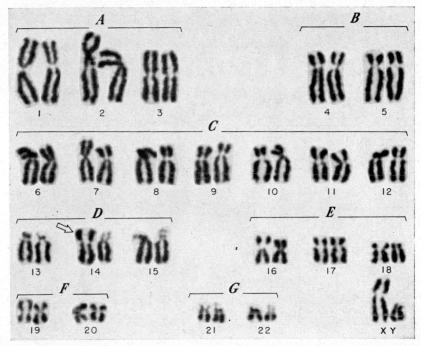

Fig. 47. Translocation Mongol. Three 21 chromosomes are present, but one has become translocated on to a D group chromosome. This can happen as a "de novo" event (as in this case), or it can happen as the result of an inherited translocation: Figs. 49, 50, 51. (*Preparation by Dr F. Sergovich*)

Although cytogeneticists may quarrel with my treatment, I will regard this as a special variety of non-disjunction; or non-disjunction to which the further process of translocation has been added. Let me emphasize again that in this type of translocation mongol the parental chromosomes are normal, just as they are in the trisomic mongol. This is most important.

Let us suppose that at gametogenesis a non-disjunction has occurred and that we have in one gamete both 21 chromosomes. Let us now suppose that the extra chromosome attaches itself, or translocates to, another

entirely different chromosome within the new gamete. Then let us
imagine fertilization of this abnormal gamete by a normal gamete with
its haploid chromosome complement. The zygote will have three 21
chromosomes, but one will not be "free". It will be less apparent as
redundancy for it is incorporated in the other chromosome (Fig. 47).
The total number of chromosomes will seem to be 46 chromosomes
only, not 47.

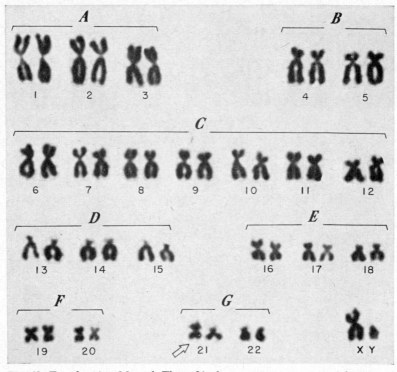

Fig. 48. Translocation Mongol. Three 21 chromosomes are present, but two are
joined by translocation. In this case it has happened as a "de novo" event. (*Preparation
by Dr F. Sergovich*)

Almost always, if not quite invariably, the extra 21 chromosome
attaches to one of the other autosomal acrocentrics. If it attaches to a
D chromosome, as in Fig. 47 the abnormality is known as a D/G translocation or (if clinical mongolism makes it by definition certain that
number 21 is involved) as a 13–15/21 translocation. If it attaches to one
of the small acrocentrics in group G (21 or 22, we cannot say which) it
is known as a G/G or 21–22/21 translocation (Fig. 48). In the 453
Manitoba mongols of Uchida there were 5 D/G and 4 G/G translocation mongols as "de novo" events. Together 2 per cent of all the mongols,

We do not know just why such "de novo" translocations happen. Insufficient cases have been studied. There seems to be just a hint that X-irradiation to the mothers' abdomen, and thus to her gonads, may be a factor. The risk of recurrence of this type of mongolism, on the basis of rather slender data, seems to be very low indeed.

Now we must consider the "inherited translocation mongol". Num-

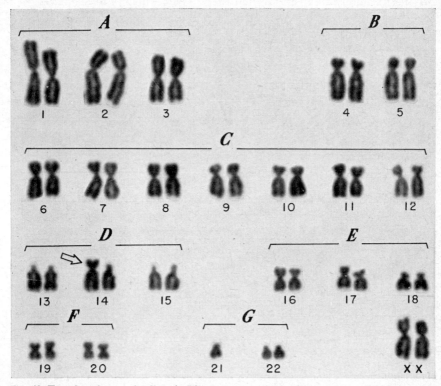

Fig. 49. Translocation-carrier Female. The possessor of this "balanced" translocation has two 21 chromosomes, but one has become translocated onto a D group chromosome: a D/G translocation. She appears to be in all ways normal, but she will have, in theory at any rate, a one-in-three chance of a mongol child: Figs. 50, 51. (*Preparation by Dr F. Sergovich*)

erically insignificant (four of 453) they are, even so, a most important group.

"Inherited Translocation" Mongols

It can happen, as we have pointed out in Chapter IV, that quite normal-seeming persons can have in their body cells one of their 21 chromosomes translocated to another, almost always to another acrocentric. Fig. 49 shows such a karyotype. Note that there is no excess nor significant deficit of chromosome material. This is a "balanced translocation". There is no reason to expect a physical deformity.

Although we have alluded to the problems posed by gametogenesis let us look at them again (Fig. 50). Let us suppose that a 21 chromosome is attached in balanced translocation to number 14. Four types of gametes can be produced. The normal 14 may migrate with the free 21. Fertilization will give a normal baby. The normal 14 may migrate to a

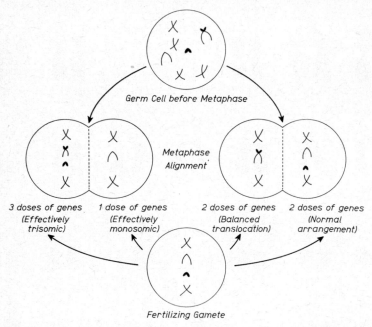

Germ Cell before Metaphase

Metaphase Alignment

3 doses of genes (*Effectively trisomic*)

1 dose of genes (*Effectively monosomic*)

2 doses of genes (*Balanced translocation*)

2 doses of genes (*Normal arrangement*)

Fertilizing Gamete

Fig. 50. *Gametogenesis in balanced translocation-carrier.* In this instance we illustrate a small acrocentric translocated on to a large acrocentric: a D/G translocation. It could be, for example, a 14/21 translocation. For simplicity only four pairs of chromosomes are shown. Four gamete possibilities exist. Four zygote possibilities can arise at fertilization: one trisomy, one monosomy, one balanced translocation-carrier and one with normal chromosome complement.

cell lacking any 21, either free or translocated. Fertilization will bring one 21 chromosome. The embryo will be monosomic and inviable. The 14/21 translocated chromosome may migrate to a gamete with no 21. Fertilization will bring another 21. The new individual will have a pair of 21 chromosomes, one free, one translocated. He will appear a normal baby but will be, like the parent, a balanced translocation carrier.

As a fourth possibility, the 14/21 chromosome may be incorporated in a gamete to which the "free" 21 has also moved. There will be both of the pair in one gamete, one free, one translocated. Fertilization will add another. There will now be three 21 chromosomes in the zygote, two free one translocated (Fig. 51). This child will be a mongol.

In the case of such a translocation-carrier parent, in theory at any rate, one child in every four conceptions will be a mongol. Since one out of every four conceptions comes to naught, one child out of every three born will be a mongol. One child in three will be quite normal in every way. One child in three will be a balanced translocation carrier

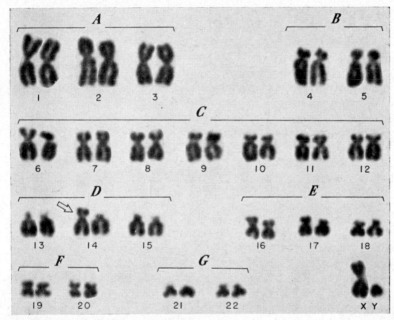

Fig. 51. Translocation Mongol, Male. The chromosome distribution is the same as in Fig. 47, but in this case the disorder has arisen because the mother is a translocation-carrier, Fig. 49, and gametogenesis has been as in Fig. 50. (*Preparation by Dr F. Sergovich*)

and will itself have, for its offspring, the same risks as had its parents for their children.

In practice it doesn't work out quite in this way. If the father is the translocation carrier very few mongol children are born; with very few exceptions, normals and carriers only are produced. The reasons are imperfectly understood—by me, I must confess. If the mother is the translocation carrier the risk of a mongol child is very high indeed. Maybe not quite as high as one-in-three (for there may be embryonic discrimination against the mongol zygote) but at least a very major risk.

It can happen in a precisely similar way that one 21 chromosome is translocated in a carrier parent on to number 22: a 21/22, G/G translocation. The parent is normal in appearance, but as in the D/G translocation-carrier parent the odds in theory are again, one mongol, one carrier, one normal child and one blighted zygote.

We have then a few mothers—and a very few—who have a one-in-three risk of mongol children, and a one-in-twelve risk that any grandchild will be a mongol. A frightening prospect indeed, but even worse has been recorded.

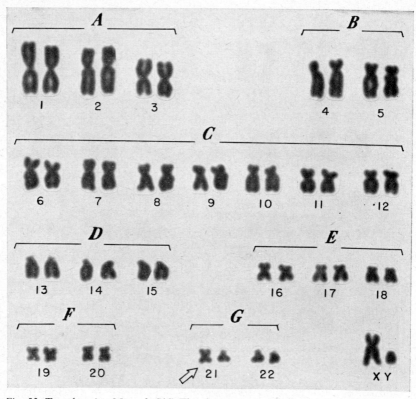

Fig. 52. Translocation Mongol, G/G. The chromosome distribution is the same as in Fig. 48, but this karyotype could have arisen because the mother was a G/G translocation-carrier. Such cases are very rare, and we have not seen one. This karyotype is an artificial assembly for demonstration purposes. (*Preparation by Dr F. Sergovich*)

Suppose that in a normal-seeming person one 21 is translocated to the other: a 21/21 translocation. What will happen at gametogenesis? Both 21 chromosomes must migrate as one. Two gamete possibilities exist: one gamete has both of the pair, the other neither. Fertilization brings another 21 (Fig. 14). Two zygote possibilities exist: a lethal monosomy or one with three of a kind, one free, two as the 21/21 translocated combination (Fig. 52). Every child born will be a mongol. It has happened.

Because the majority of mongols are born to older mothers, and are mongols because of non-disjunction of an ageing ovum, it follows that it is among young mothers that such other mechanisms as inherited translocation mongolism are most likely to be found. Certainly the young mother may suffer the chance mishap of non-disjunction but it is among the young mothers that the high risk cases should be sought. The matter is important when one has to manage the mongol and to advise his parents.

Management of the Child with Mongolism

The doctor who deals with the problems of a mongol child faces more than the problems of that child alone. The whole family needs help; none more so than the distraught parents upon whom this tragedy has fallen. Much delicacy of rapport is needed if the disaster is to be mitigated and the poor parents guided to accept in the best possible way the misfortune that has come upon them. "In one short hour all their hopes, dreams, and plans are shattered." They will suffer agonies of disbelief, guilt and rejection, torn as they will be between a love which has been nine months in preparation and an unwillingness to accept so imperfect a baby.

Faced with a mother with her newborn baby, what should the doctor do if he suspects that the baby is a mongol. Should he say nothing until time proclaims his apparent lack of diagnostic acumen, or should he straightaway voice his suspicion. It is not easy, but I believe he should be brave, but brave with caution.

The average practitioner will see few mongol babies, and he may well be uncertain of the diagnosis. If he works in a centre (and most do not) where chromosome studies can be done he can arrange for a blood lymphocyte culture to be done without the mother's knowledge. If it is normal, he can secretly rejoice and no harm is done. If the diagnosis is proved in two or three days he will have to face the parents telling them of the certain diagnosis. Unfortunately in the immediate newborn period dermatoglyphic patterns are too small and indistinct to be interpreted with any certainty, even by an expert.

If a specialist pædiatrician, who may have seen many mongol babies, is at hand, let him be consulted unknown to the parents. The diagnosis may then be confirmed, refuted, or even still in doubt. If the specialist agrees with the suspicion, something must be said; if he does not, it is probably best to invent some reason, other than a question of a disorder involving mental retardation, for his visit. If mental retardation has been questioned, even with re-assurance, the parents will watch and wonder for months, and years. If doubt remains after the consultation, say nothing. Time will make the issue clear.

I have heard it taught that the father of the baby, or perhaps some other relative, only should hear the news and that the knowledge should be kept from the mother. What unrealistic advice! What a secret this would be for a husband or other relative to keep from the proud and unsuspecting mother with her newborn baby. No, both parents must be told at one time, together, that all is not well. It is a dismal task requiring the greatest tact and sympathy. But it is better, I find, that it be done as soon as possible. Delay cannot make matters any better.

If there has been doubt at first, and nothing has been said, wait until you are certain. It is often as well then to refer the baby for another opinion. Perhaps you would prefer that the specialist has the unpleasant task of breaking the news. When making a referral please let the specialist know how much the mother knows of why consultation is sought; let him know how much you would like him to tell the mother. A consultation can be well worthwhile. This author in his younger days made a mistake and diagnosed mongolism in a normal newborn baby. The repercussions of such an error are not easily forgotten. Seek confirmation, be sure, and then tell the truth. It is better so.

One must explain that this is a rare disease, a chance mishap (it could happen to oneself) in which an egg cell has split unequally so that factors for inheritance have become unbalanced. There is an excess of factors that determine development and growth. Too many orders and instructions have led to confusion in the body and to abnormal growth. One must be sure that it is understood that neither parent is to blame. This is not due to disease in either parent nor to anything done or left undone during the pregnancy. It is a chance mishap. Sometimes in-laws need to be told this too!

It is perhaps wise not to emphasize too much the relation to maternal age once the misfortune has come about lest guilt be felt at having a baby at an older age. To risk such guilt can now do no good.

One must be frank and say that this baby, loveable though he may be, will be a simple soul. He will be happy, cheerful and content but never be able to attend a normal school, or in later years be fully self-supporting. He, or she, will not marry and have children.

He will walk, but be late in doing so. He will talk but will be slow and simple in his use of words. He will become clean but this may take a little longer than usual. He may attend a day school for retarded children if one be near at hand; if not, he may have to go away to a residential school for retarded children. As he gets older he may be happier among those of his own kind.

Unless he has congenital heart disease his health in general will be good though upper respiratory infections may be a problem. Apart from heart disease, other congenital abnormalities are not usual. If some disease or abnormality requires treatment or surgery the question often arises: should one treat a mongol. If so, how much? I have come to believe that one cannot stand idly by (and ask nurses to stand more closely idly by) and let the child die or suffer untreated. I have come to believe that one must treat the mongol just like any other child.

In my view one must tell the parents to be frank with their relatives and friends. They must be open about their misfortune. This is not a matter for shame or for concealment. Imagine the heartache of a mother who knows the facts but tries to respond in cheerful terms to kind and well-meaning enquiries about her new baby. She must make the facts known to her other children and to her friends and neighbours. If she does not, she will avoid meeting them and become a recluse.

A mongol baby was referred to me from a distance. The father was a scientist who knew about chromosomes and he asked that cyto-genetic studies be made to confirm the diagnosis. The blood was taken for culture and the baby was taken home. In a few days the diagnosis was confirmed and I wrote to the parents expressing my sorrow that the test showed beyond doubt that their baby was a mongol. The father had my letter copied and sent it to his friends and relatives. This was cold-blooded, but he had the right idea. When the truth is out, there is no more to be said.

What can be done for the child with mongolism? The truth must be stated. There is no cure. This must be said quite firmly. Desperate parents otherwise may take the child from doctor to doctor, from charlatan, sometimes, to charlatan, from continent to continent seeking what does not exist. Disappointment only, and financial loss, will be their rewards. One must make the best of this child as he is, not seek the unobtainable.

It is now generally believed that the best can be made of the potential of this child if he is kept at home, loved by his parents and his sibs, taught and played with in a home environment—for some years at any rate. If the parents can accept him and his disease he should be kept at home for several years. Most parents can and will. He will not be difficult to handle.

When he reaches school age new problems arise. Ideally he should be kept at home for some years yet, attending a day school for retarded children. If there is no such school he may be kept at home, or he may go away to a residential hospital school so that the best may be made of his potential. The attitude of the family and the environment will probably decide this issue.

He will not become self-supporting, and the parents cannot look after him for ever. Moreover they are likely to be elderly and perhaps by adult life he will be alone. Most mongols come, if only for this reason, into institutional care in time. Circumstances, of course, alter cases but in the society from which I write the advice is to keep the child with mongolism at home, if only for a few years. The parents will then feel that they have done their best.

C.D.   H

What of the other children? Will the mongol in their midst harm them? If the neighbours and their children know the facts, if their playmates know the truth, if the parents of the mongol feel no shame nor blame, no harm, I think, will come to the sibs of the mongol child. Knowledge of the facts will bring acceptance and compassion. Secrecy will engender taunts and ridicule.

Genetic Counselling in Mongolism

Genetic counselling is not concerned solely with risk facts and figures. It embraces an explanation of the cause of the disease. Guilt must be dispelled and recrimination between spouses, and sometimes in-laws, dissipated. The genetic counsellor must concern himself with these things while remembering that it is not his function to instruct people as to what they must or must not do in the matter of having children. Only parents know how much they are prepared to risk to attain, maybe, their heart's desires.

What are the risk figures and risk facts? What are the chances that any couple may have a mongol child—or another mongol child? What are the risks of recurrence of mongolism?

A mother who has no mongol child and no mongols among relatives has a risk related to her age (Fig. 37). One chance, let us say, in 2000–3000 at 25, one in 200 at 35, perhaps as high as one in 40 at age 40 years and over. These are rough figures and empiric figures, but they will suffice.

When one has to advise a mother with a mongol child on the risk of another mongol, one is on less sure ground. At the hazard of being too dogmatic, let us see just what can be said.

If the mother is over 35 at the birth of her first mongol, it is almost certain that that mongol was conceived of the chance mishap of non-disjunction due to abnormal meiotic segregation of an ageing ovum. Although we do not know why, there is evidence that even non-disjunction mongolism tends to weak familiality. There is a slightly increased risk, beyond the risk for anyone, that such non-disjunction might occur again. The increased risk is not very great, but it may be about a four-fold increase of the age-dependent risk as shown in Fig. 37. Let us say, then, at 25 a risk of 1 : 500 for recurrence, at 35 a risk of 1 : 50, perhaps at age 40 a risk of 1 : 10. Such an estimate is the best that we can do in our imperfect state of knowledge.

If the mother is young, and the younger the more is this so, it becomes less likely that non-disjunction is the mechanism; more likely that there is some other cause. It is true that at all ages non-disjunction mongols greatly out-number those due to translocation, but it is among young mothers that translocation must especially be sought.

In the mother of, say, 35 and under, chromosome studies if possible should be done. Nowadays many laboratories are able to give this service, either by directly taking blood, setting up cultures and making slides for karyotype analysis or, using such kits as those put out by Difco, by starting the culture of the cells and making slides locally, to be sent to a centre for analysis. If a centre for chromosome analysis is only a day or two away "mail order" chromosome studies may be successful. Uchida suggests that 10 ml. of blood be taken in a heparinized syringe and added to 0·5 ml. of heparin in a sterile tube. The sample now stands at room temperature for between three and six hours. The supernatant plasma is removed and transferred to a bottle. A drop or two of the sedimented red cells are added together with phytohaemagglutinin.* The whole is then sent to a cytogenetics laboratory, air-mail, special delivery, not at weekends.

Studies of the mongol should first be made. If he is shown to be of regular trisomic type, he is a non-disjunction mongol and the fourfold-the-age dependent rule is valid. If he is a translocation mongol both parents should be checked. If their chromosomes are normal, the mongol is an example of "de novo" translocation and the risk of recurrence is very slight indeed; perhaps almost negligible.

But one or other of the parents may, while themselves normal, have an abnormal karyotype. Where a mongol child is born by inherited translocation it is almost always the mother who is the translocation-carrier. Carrier fathers only very rarely have mongol children. The mother, then, may be a balanced translocation-carrier; perhaps, as in Fig. 49, a D/G translocation-carrier.

Should this be so, the risk of recurrence is very high indeed; maybe as high as theory would expect; that is to say, one chance in every three children. Maybe it will be something less than that, but the risk will be high enough that the couple must be advised to think carefully before having additions to the family.

Mr and Mrs D. . . . , both under 30, had two children. The third was a mongol. Because of their ages this mongol child was tested. He was a D/G translocation mongol (Fig. 51). Mrs D . . . was shown to be a balanced D/G translocation-carrier (Fig. 49). Her eldest child, a boy, was also a balanced carrier. Her daughter had normal chromosomes. Her risks at gametogenesis had been (and by chance had worked out thus) as shown in Fig. 50.

Our advice was this. The risk of another mongol was for Mrs D . . . perhaps as high as 1 : 3; for another carrier, also as high as 1 : 3. Only she knew what so high a risk meant to her. She wanted another child, but she adopted one.

Her oldest son, also a carrier will almost certainly not have mongol children. Male carriers very, very rarely do. There seems to be selection against a sperm bearing an extra load of chromosome material. Male

*Can be supplied by Burroughs Wellcome and Company (branches throughout the world). Add. 5 ml. of sterile pyrogen per water to each unit of phytohaemagglutinin and use 0·1 ml. to each ml. of plasma.

carriers have normal and carrier children only, in roughly equal numbers.

Now, if he has male children about half will be, like him, translocation-carriers. Those carriers will, like him, be spared from having mongol children but will, like him, have carriers and normals in equal numbers.

If, on the other hand, this son of Mrs D . . . has female children, half may be D/G translocation-carriers. They, being female, will have a risk maybe as high as 1 : 3 of having mongol children. Mrs D . . . in this way has a 1 : 12 chance of having mongol great-grandchildren through her eldest son.

Mrs D . . . had a married sister who at the time of this investigation was expecting her first child. We did not feel it useful or kind at that point to tell her that she could be at risk of having a mongol child soon to be born. The baby was normal. This sister of Mrs D . . . was tested and found also to be a D/G carrier. She had been lucky. She has been advised accordingly.

Intra-Uterine Diagnosis, Amniocentesis

Could we have tested that baby before it was born? The answer is, yes, we could. Exfoliated cells from an unborn baby can now be grown with 70 per cent success in tissue culture. We are not sure just where those cells, suspended in the amniotic fluid, have come from, but they are the baby's cells. They will grow, and karyotypes can be made.

This new technique raises most difficult legal and moral issues. Suppose the unborn baby had been tested and found to be a D/G trans-location mongol; what would one do? In most societies the termination of such a pregnancy is, at the best, an illegal operation; at the worst it is murder. Science has outrun the law.

Even though the law in many societies would not countenance abortion of even an undoubtedly abnormal foetus, in some countries such an abortion could legally be done. The indications for amniotic tap and ante-natal diagnosis might be these: a balanced translocation in a mother where one can be certain that in her (and so in the baby) the site of the translocation can be recognized, and a translocation mongol distinguished from a normal baby; a mother of over 35 who already has one mongol child; a mother of over 40 who is beside herself with anxiety because she knows what the risk might be. She can be reassured that all is well or—if the law allows, aborted. Here are new forensic problems to which public opinion will soon demand solution. One thing seems certain as things stand at present. It would be cruel indeed to offer a mother ante-natal diagnosis unless one was prepared, law or no law, to procure abortion if her baby were shown to be defective.

Chapter VIII
Other Autosomal Abnormalities

One might imagine that since such a stereotyped abnormality as mongolism is invariably associated with a chromosome anomaly, other comparable associations might be found. One might perhaps expect to see a chromosome defect in achondroplasia, anencephaly, amaurotic family idiocy, or phenylketonuria, to name but a few that have been investigated in this respect. Such is not the case. Only quite rarely, except in mongolism and the sex chromosome anomalies, is a chromosome anomaly regularly found with congenital deformity or defect.

It is likely that excess or deficit of most of the chromosomes produce such profound effects that the development of the embryo ceases at an early stage and that the product of conception is reabsorbed unrecognized as a pregnancy. No doubt there are minute abnormalities of the chromosomes in many defects, but it seems that they are so subtle that they cannot be seen by our crude methods. Time and refinements surely will change that.

In the past few years we have come to recognize, in addition to mongolism, a few stereotyped disorders, some of them quite rare, with constant chromosome disorder. Certain features, presumably of the most vulnerable systems, tend to be seen in common. Mental retardation is always found, except in the sex chromosome anomalies. Low birth weight is almost universal. Abnormality of development of the first visceral arch is common. Low set and abnormally developed ears are often found, as are pre-auricular pits, accessory auricles or skin tags. Micrognathia is very common. Congenital heart disease and cleft lip or palate are usual.

The D_1-Trisomy Syndrome

This is a rare disease in the living infant. Even now only a few dozen cases are on record, but most people interested in such things have recognized one or two. Perhaps one in every five thousand babies born has this deformity. The abnormalities are so constant that the diagnosis can often be made at birth. The syndrome, first described by Bartholin in 1657, was re-defined by Patau in 1960. Sometimes the disorder is known as Patau's syndrome.

The baby is frail, puny, and microcephalic. There may be deformities of the scalp or skull and there is invariably cleft lip or palate. These are the hallmarks of the condition. Microphthalmus or anophthalmus are very common, as are diffuse capillary haemangiomas. Very often rudimentary digits are found on hands and feet. The fingers often are fixed in flexion. The whole appearance is unmistakable (Fig. 53).

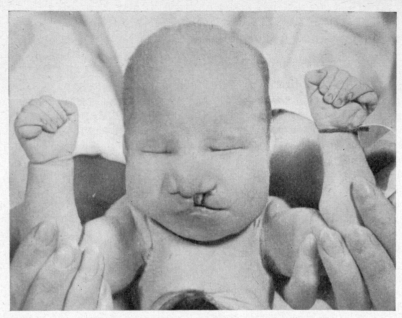

Fig. 53. D₁ Trisomy Syndrome. The extra digits are unusually well developed in this case. This was not a living patient, but was found in the Dept. of Anatomy of The University of Western Ontario having been preserved for 30 years! The typical features leave no doubt as to the diagnosis. (*Courtesy of Prof. M. L. Barr*)

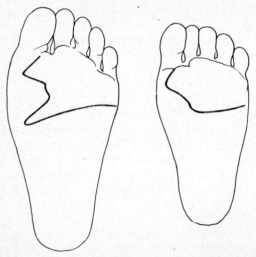

Fig. 54. D₁ Trisomy Syndrome: dermal ridge pattern on soles. The characteristic Fibular Arch of two cases is shown in outline. (*H. C. Soltan and Irene Uchida, Evaluation of Dermatoglyphics in Medical Genetics, Pediat. Clin. N. Amer. 10(2), May 1963, W. B. Saunders Co, Philadelphia*)

Congenital heart deformity is common. Usually it is a ventricular septal defect but there may be dextrocardia and other lesions of wide variety. Hydronephrosis, renal cysts, abnormal lobulation of lungs, septate uterus and accessory spleens have commonly been found. In early infancy the embryonic haemoglobin, Gower-2, may be found. In those that survive a year or two the foetal haemoglobin-F persists beyond the time when normally it disappears.

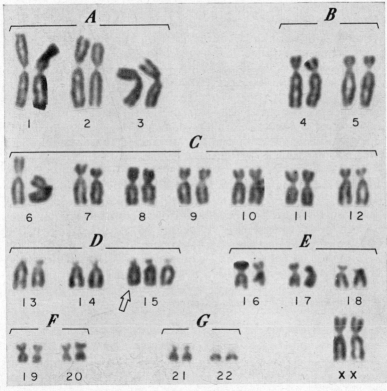

Fig. 55. Trisomy of one of the chromosomes in Group D. One cannot say which, for the D group chromosomes cannot be distinguished. (*Preparation by Dr H. Carr*)

The dermal ridge patterns are abnormal. Although the digital patterns are not unusual, the axis triradius is in a very high, extremely distal, position; the atd angle is obtuse. Extra patterns are common on thenar and hypothenar eminences. Simian palm creases are often seen. On the hallucal area of the foot there may be a diagnostic pattern, a S-shaped fibular arch (Fig. 54). Such a pattern made the diagnosis in the baby in Fig. 53, although it had been preserved as a museum specimen for thirty years.

These babies usually live but a few days or weeks. Occasionally one will live two or three years. If they do, severe mental defect is the rule. At autopsy other defects are found. There is abnormal development of the frontal region of the brain and of the olfactory lobes. The corpus callosum is often absent and there may be hypoplasia of the cerebellum. The condition of the brain may be referred to as "arrhinencephaly".

Trisomy of one of the D group chromosomes is the essential feature (Fig. 55). One cannot say whether it is pair 13, 14, or 15 that is in triplicate, for these pairs cannot be distinguished by their size or shape. It is possible, but by now rather unlikely, that two other D-trisomy syndromes await description. It is for this reason that the syndrome we have described is often called the D_1 syndrome: the first to be described.

It is believed that the usual mechanism for production of this trisomy is non-disjunction of the maternal gamete for, as in mongolism, there is a significant relation to maternal age. But as in mongolism, non-disjunction is not the only mechanism. In our series of 2159 newborn babies we found one example of this syndrome. The mother was a D/D translocation-carrier. Both of one pair of D group chromosomes had migrated into one gamete. Fertilization had added another. There was, effectively, trisomy of a D group though there were, in all, only 46 chromosomes; a situation comparable to that shown for mongolism in Fig. 52.

It is possible that the D-syndrome is potentially quite common but that the abnormal conceptus is commonly miscarried. Our neonatal survey revealed one translocation D-syndrome and one balanced D/D translocation-carrier baby (both of whose mothers were D/D balanced carriers). In 483 random adults Court Brown found one woman who was a mosaic of normal and D/D translocation cells. Carr in his 227 aborted foetuses found six D group trisomics.

The E-Trisomy Syndrome

This disorder is not so very rare, though it is less common than mongolism. Many cases are on record, and it has been estimated that perhaps one in every 2000 babies has this disease. I have myself seen several examples of this syndrome in the last five years or so. Carr found nine E-trisomics in his 227 aborted products of conception.

The babies are thin, frail, and puny. They fail to thrive and early death is usual.

Two have survived to three and ten years of age. Both were very severely retarded mentally.

The occiput is prominent and the ears low set and malformed. The chin is receding but the eyes rather protruding. Brain deformity seems to be variable; some have reported no gross or visible defect, others have noted hypoplasia of the cerebellum or absence of the corpus callosum.

One of the most striking features of these babies is their rigidity. Their limbs, held in flexion, scarcely can be moved. The reflexes, however, do not seem to be increased. The fingers are tightly flexed at the metacarpophalangeal joints and are rigidly fixed across the palm. The index finger is strangely deviated to the ulnar side crossing backward over the third digit. The fingers can hardly be extended, even by quite strong force (Fig. 56).

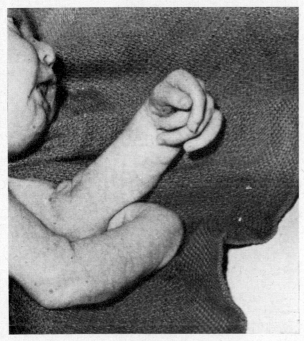

Fig. 56. E Syndrome (sometimes called without equivocation Trisomy-18). The fingers are rigidly flexed and the index finger crosses over the third digit.

The feet are often curious. The big toe may be short and dorsiflexed, or there may be "rocker-bottom" feet. The sole may be convex and the heel prominent, giving an appearance like the runners of a rocking-chair. The baby illustrated in Fig. 57 was diagnosed at a glance—from the feet protruding from the bed covers.

There may be other malformations. The sternum is often short. Heart defects and renal deformities are common; so too are meningo-myelocoeles and Meckel's diverticula. Inguinal, lumbar and umbilical hernias are also often found.

It is not easy to examine the dermal ridge patterns for the fingers are firmly fixed across the palm. The axis triradius is in a very distal position.

Fifty per cent of cases have a transverse palmar crease. A single fifth digit crease is found in nearly a quarter of the cases. There is often no pattern on the hallux, only an "open-field". It is the digital patterns, however, that are startling. Very many arches are found. In 30 per cent of cases all fingers have arches and this is unheard of in normal persons. In other cases six or more arches are to be found. Fifteen patients with

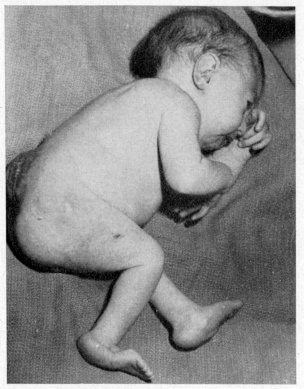

Fig. 57. E Syndrome. Note especially the "rocker-bottom" feet, the micrognathia, the prominent occiput and, in this case, a meningomyelocoele.

this syndrome together amassed 128 arches on their 150 digits. There are likewise many arches on the toes.

The essential chromosome abnormality is trisomy in group E. One cannot say for sure which pair is represented in triplicate, but it is almost certainly not pair 16. Opinion generally seems to favour 18 as the deviant pair, and the condition is sometimes referred to without equivocation as trisomy-18 (Fig. 58).

Again it seems likely that non-disjunction in the maternal gamete is the cause, for 52 per cent of mothers in one study were over 35 years of age compared with 10 per cent for the mothers of normal babies. Like mongolism and trisomy-D, trisomy-E seems to be age-dependent but other mechanisms could be responsible. No doubt there could be iso-chromosome formation increasing, or at least unbalancing, the load of gene material of chromosome 18. No doubt a trisomy in effect could be produced by a translocation-carrier parent.

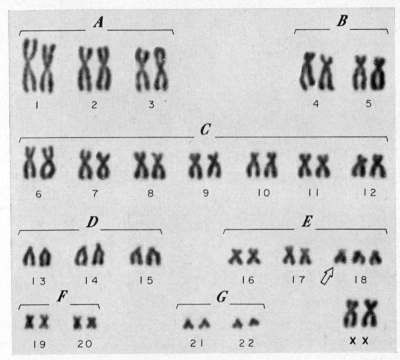

Fig. 58. Karyotype of E Trisomy Syndrome showing triple representation of chromosome number 18. (*Preparation by Dr D. H. Carr*)

It does not seem as though very many trisomy-18 conceptions are cast out as miscarriage. In 227 abortions Carr found nine E-trisomics, but six were trisomic for number 16.

Chromosome 18 Deletions, "Carp-Mouth" Syndrome

Of late deletion of part of the long arm of chromosome 18 has been judged to cause a specific syndrome though only some 20 cases are on record. It has been called by some the "Carp-Mouth" Syndrome (Fig. 59a, b).

The birth weight is low, mental retardation is severe. The head is small, the ears are low with prominent helix and anti-helix; the chin

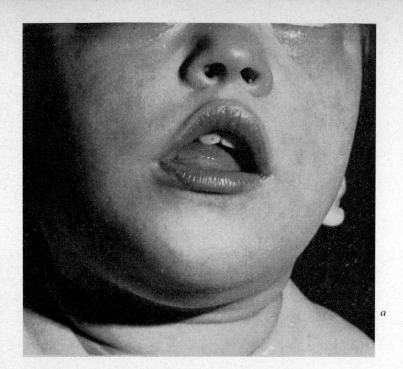

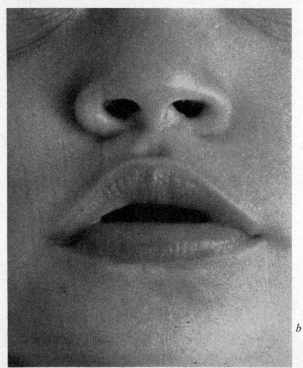

Fig. 59a and b. The "carp-mouth" associated with deletion of part of the long arms of chromosome 18. (*Kindly supplied by Dr J. D. Blair, Metropolitan General Hospital, Cleveland, Ohio*)

tends to be large but the nose is small. The columella of the upper lip is absent and the mouth is somewhat fish-like. The hands are small, the fingers tapered and the thumbs set back in the hand towards the wrist. The fingers bear an increased frequency of whorls. In males there may be hypospadias; the testes are not usually descended. The picture

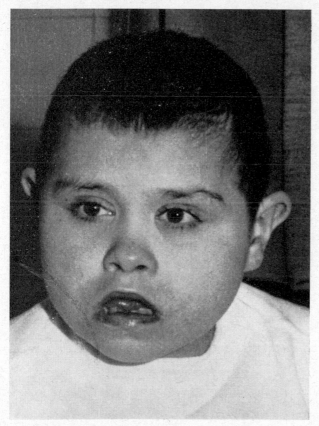

Fig. 60. Syndrome of deletion of part of the long arms of chromosome 18. This is a different case from Fig. 59a and b, but note that the mouth is similar. (*Kindly supplied by Dr F. Sergovich*)

perhaps is not clinically very specific (Fig. 60) but some claim clinical recognition. The karyotype shows loss of about half of the long arms of the 18 chromosome (Fig. 61).

Deletion of the short arms of the 18 chromosome has been reported several times. Although the clinical picture is something less than specific, it is said that next to the "Cat-Cry" this is the most common of the autosome deletions. Low birth weight and mental retardation seem to be the rule. Growth failure is usual. There may be hyperteliorism, squint, and a webbed neck; cebocephaly (single nostril and nasal atresia), cyclops and, perhaps, immune globulin IgA deficiency may add specificity to an otherwise rather non-specific picture.

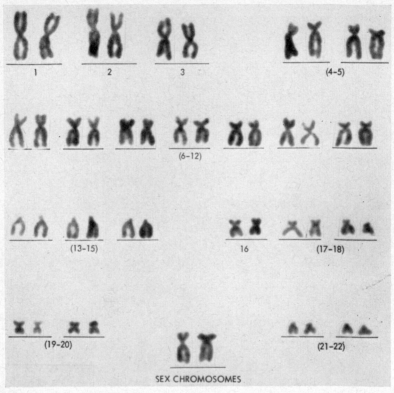

Fig. 61. Karyotype of "Carp-mouth Syndrome" showing deletion of part of the long arms of chromosome 18. (*Preparation kindly supplied by Dr J. D. Blair, The Metropolitan General Hospital, Cleveland, Ohio*)

Cat-Cry Syndrome, Cri-du-Chat

After the syndrome of D and E trisomy were described it hardly seemed likely that any other syndrome of chromosome anomaly would be described with any degree of regularity or ease of recognition, but in 1964 Lejeune described La Maladie du Cri-du-Chat. It is not rare.

These babies, who may survive quite well, exhibit, at least in early infancy, a clear-cut picture. There is a round moon-face (Fig. 62), microcephaly, hyperteliorism and low birth weight. There may be epicanthic folds and micrognathia. The dermal patterns are not too unusual though transverse palmar creases are usual and the axis triradius may be distal.

It is the cry that is striking. It is quite weird. It is a plaintive high-pitched wail, weak, and with a hint of stridor. It really does sound like the mewing of a kitten. At one time when we had such a baby in our nurseries a cleaning-woman hearing the cry spent some time searching

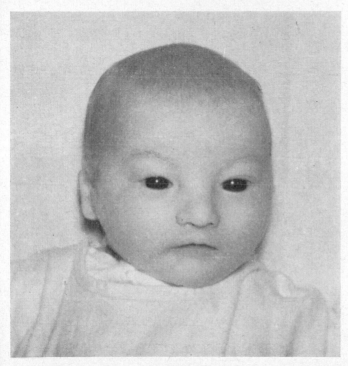

Fig. 62. David G: Cat-cry Syndrome. Age four days. This picture, taken before it was realized that he was abnormal, was obtained from a routine neonatal identification photograph. (*Supplied by The City General Hospital, Chatham, Ontario*)

for the stray kitten! This cry results from laryngomalacia, with narrow vocal cords and a curved epiglottis. On phonation there is an air-leak at the posterior commissure and the strange cry comes from the approximated cords in front. As these babies grow older this feature disappears. While they tend to have stridor and repeated upper respiratory infections the cry is no longer distinctive; nor, perhaps, is the facial appearance. They come to look much like other retarded children (Fig. 63). There is perhaps one distinctive feature that was present in two cases seen by myself and in others illustrated in the literature: a flat sessile nodule, two or three millimetres in diameter, a centimetre or so in front of each ear.

The chromosome disorder is a deletion. Part of the short arm of a B group chromosome is missing. It is believed to be B5 (Fig. 64). In

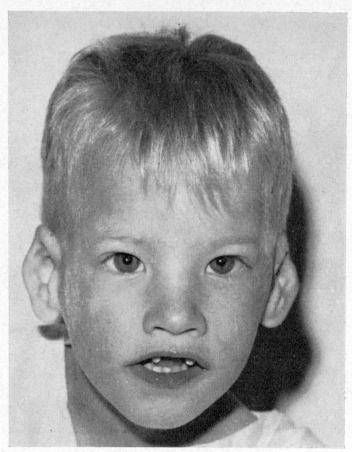

Fig. 63. David G: Cat-cry Syndrome. This is the same child as in Fig. 62. He is now aged four years. Note that the round face is no longer a feature. He has no speech and is severely retarded, but his cry is not now remarkable.

general it seems that the deletion comes about as a chance mishap, a break and then a loss at anaphase. One case of mine shows how this might come about.

Nancy M. is a typical case of Cri-du-Chat. Part of the short arm of one B5 is missing. Her father is normal phenotypically, but his karyotype is quite unusual. One of his B5 chromosomes has a long constriction in the short arms. Part of each short arm is carried on a stalk. At gametogenesis these stalks have broken and the distal fragment has become lost.

This is not the only way that deletion could occur. A parent could be a balanced translocation-carrier. Part of the short arm of B5 could be attached to another chromosome. There could be a balanced short-arm B5 translocation. At gametogenesis the B5 chromosome with the deleted

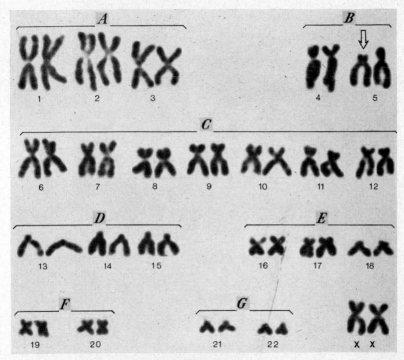

Fig. 64. Karyotype of the "Cat-cry Syndrome" showing deletion of part of the short arm of one of the B group chromosomes, presumed to be B5. (*Preparation by Cytogenetics Laboratory, Victoria Hospital, London, Ontario*)

arm could migrate into a gamete without the chromosome that bears the translocated fragment. Fertilization would add a normal B5. The zygote would become a cat-cry baby. This has happened.

   Although B5 and B4 look very similar they can, so it is claimed, be distinguished by autoradiography (see Chapter III, Special Techniques). Deletion of B4 has been identified and associated with a combination of low birth weight at term, exophalmos, broad and beaked nose, inguinal hernias, undescended testes, hypospadias—but with a normal cry.

Miscellaneous

As we have said, and seen, there are rather few defects with deformities that can with any regularity be blamed on autosomal chromosome anomaly. There are only four occurring more than exceptionally: mongolism, trisomy-D, trisomy-E, and the cat-cry syndrome.

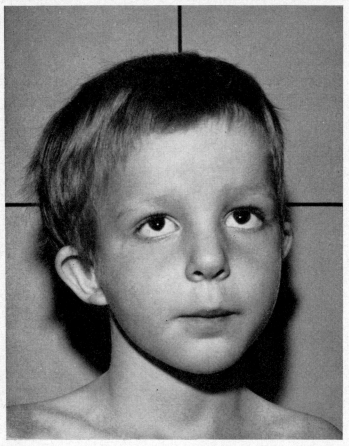

Fig. 65. An unusual case. Slight degree of mental retardation only, congenital heart disease and unusual appearance. Karyotype shows trisomy of a G group chromosome, believed to be number 22. Trisomy 22 is not a syndrome that can be recognized by specific features. (*Kindly supplied by Dr W. Langdon, London, Ontario*)

The literature abounds with fancied associations and unique events. To take examples from personal experience: Fig. 65 shows a retarded girl of odd appearance. She has a heart deformity, a simian crease and malformed ears. Her karyotype alone would lead one to suppose that she is a mongol. Clearly she is not, although she is trisomic for what appears to be a G group chromosome. We believe that she is a 22 trisomy; one of the very, very few.

One writer reported a chromosome anomaly in giant haemangioma with thrombocytopaenia. In a case of ours no such anomaly was found. In a case of ours of the oral-facial-digital syndrome of Papillon-Leage we found no chromosome anomaly though such has been found in another case of that disorder. Several reports have been made of various chromosome anomalies of the C group chromosomes (perhaps C11) in Cornelia de Lange's syndrome. Cases of ours have shown no chromosome anomaly.

A small boy was referred for suspected retardation. His I.Q. was indeed low and he had a severe hearing loss. His appearance was odd; his face was not unlike that of a ventriloquist's mannikin. He had stiff fingers and a hammer toe. Chromosome study of his lymphocytes was normal. Because his dermal patterns were quite unusual, further studies were done. Culture of skin fibroblasts showed trisomy of a C group chromosome. He is a mosaic for a C group trisomy. Is he a mosaic for de Lange's syndrome? His face, although he does not have bushy eyebrows or long eyelashes, is certainly suggestive.

The specialized literature, and even nowadays the more general journals, appear to welcome such reports. The inconstant patterns and innumerable variations leave one confused.

What is the status of the "Big-Thumb" syndrome of Rubenstein-Taybi, with its mental retardation, beaked nose, high triradii, increased arches and hypothenar loops. The thumbs and toes are very broad; the face somewhat like mongolism. Is it a chromosome disorder; or is it not? Some would contend that it represents a very slight degree of the D-syndrome: that there is partial trisomy-D, translocated to another chromosome, maybe number 16.

Fanconi's Anaemia (Pancytopaenia, bone defects and growth failure), Bloom's Syndrome (Telangiectatic erythema, growth failure, and strange "sharp" features) and Ataxia Telangiectasia (cerebellar disturbance, telangiectasia and thymic immunological incompetence) are an intriguing trio. All are associated with chromosome breaks and all, like mongolism, show a propensity to leukaemia.

Then what is the relationship of the chromosome disorders to leukaemia at all? Where does that small residual fragment of chromosome 21, the Philadelphia Chromosome, fit in? It is present in the blood lymphocyte cultures of those with chronic myeloid leukaemia. Is it the cause? Is it the result of the leukaemia? It has been found before the leukaemia became evident. Had the leukaemia started at that point? Can we say that chronic myeloid leukaemia is a chromosome disorder? Perhaps we can.

Chapter IX
Sex Chromosomes, Reprise

Since in our discussions of the sex chromosome anomalies we will be using the terms "Male" and "Female" we must consider what those terms mean. It is not so easy as it might seem.

When we use those terms we refer to the "phenotypic sex", and the phenotypic sex describes what the person looks like, irrespective of what the gonads may be or what chromosome complement exists. A male is one who looks, to the observer of the external body form, like a boy or man. He has a penis and a scrotum. A female, in our terms of reference, looks like a girl or woman. There is a common urogenital cleft (Fig. 66). The ability to produce sperm or ova, to menstruate or to be fertile are irrelevant to our definition.

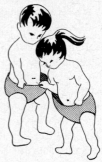

There IS a difference !

Fig. 66. Genital Sex. (*Drawn by Miss Leonie Duncan, University of Western Ontario Art Service. Adapted from a beer mat in the possession of Prof. M. L. Barr*)

Because of the rather odd economy of nature that uses the same apparatus for both reproduction and urination (an economy that might be explained by the supposition that passages that are relatively rarely used might benefit from frequent flushings), sex in our terms of reference determines what toilet facilities are to be used. We might almost say that a female is one who sits with the ladies; a male one who stands with the gentlemen. The point is not made frivolously, for it is pertinent to consider what society, denied a view of the external genitalia, might consider criteria of "male" and "female". Women may wear clothes traditionally an attribute of males. Males may dress their hair in manners that tradition ascribes to females. Females indulge in activities that at other periods in history were considered the prerogatives of males. No doubt by some subtle means the young people of today make no mistakes when they select their companions in mating situations, but surely in the last analysis society at large will judge sex by whether the individual uses the "Ladies" or the "Gents" (Fig. 67). Perhaps in deciding phenotypic sex the call of nature is the moment of truth. The potentiality to use the one facility or the other must strongly be borne in mind in deciding the upbringing, and thus the psychic gender of a child.

It would be unrealistic, and most unkind, to bring up a child as male simply because his chromosome complement was XY and his gonads

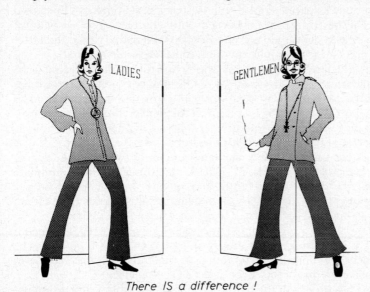

There *IS* a difference !

Fig. 67. Social Sex. (*Drawn by Miss Leonie Duncan, University of Western Ontario Art Service*)

testes on microscopic examination if, in the nude, he looked like a girl and was unable to use a male urinal.

Sexuality is psychologically undifferentiated at birth. It becomes differentiated increasingly with life experience and that, for the most part is determined by the light in which the child is regarded by his parents, his peers and by society. Gender imprinting begins at about one year; for the most part the gender role is fixed by two and one half years. Beyond that time most careful consideration must be given to the psychic turmoil that may result from late change of role. Only perhaps reproductive potential in a role different to that which has been assigned justifies a change. Better a well-adjusted gender role discordant with genetic sex than mental anguish to satisfy the demands of scientific tidiness.

Sex Determination

Although the factors determining sex have been briefly discussed in Chapter I, a re-statement may be helpful here.

Sex is determined by inductor substances that develop in the zygote under the influence of genetic constitution. The target for these inductors, whatever they may be, is the undifferentiated gonad with its outer cortex and inner medulla. If the father transmits to the zygote a Y chromosome, the medulla will develop preferentially, and a testis will form. That testis in its turn will produce two, maybe more, hormonal secretions, one a steroid similar to testosterone, the other a non-steroid substance. The former is concerned with stimulation of growth of Wolffian duct system (that becomes the vas and epididymis); the latter with suppression of the mullerian ducts (the utero-vaginal canal).

A testis will develop and maleness will (with a notable exception to be discussed later) result, irrespective of the number of X chromosomes that may be superadded by chromosomal error. On the other hand, if by error more than one Y is incorporated in the chromosome constitution of the zygote there is no greater than normal testis development: no greater degree of sexual development or prowess.

If the father transmits an X chromosome to the zygote, if the zygote is XX, inductor substances of genetic determination will stimulate growth of the cortex of the embryonic gonad and there will be un-inhibited growth of the Mullerian system but no stimulus to Wolffian duct development. The latter will wither away to a mere remnant.

In the event that a sex chromosome is lost to the normal complement, XY or XX, there could be, in theory at least, YO and XO zygotes. The complement YO appears to be lethal to the embryo; none have ever been observed. What of the effect of the XO complement?

As Carr has observed, the living XO baby represents a tiny residue of the many that are conceived. XO is highly lethal to the fœtus. As he has said, a Y chromosome (or an X) protects the foetus from intra-uterine death. Unless two XX chromosomes are present there is a failure to maintain normal ovarian development. According to the study of Singh in this centre, the ovaries seem to start off quite well. In the XO early embryo the ovaries seem normal, germ cells migrate to the gonadal ridge; all seems to be well—at first. Then things go wrong. The ovaries, especially the germ cells, atrophy, and by the time of birth (and to an increasing degree as time goes on) the ovaries are replaced by mere fibrous streaks: "streak ovaries", as they are called.

The ovary, however, is not essential for development of female ducts and female external genitalia. If the foetal testis is removed early female genitalia likewise will develop. The tendency is to female phenotype unless a Y chromosome is present to evoke a testis that in its turn will induce masculinity and repress female development. The Y chromosome then is the active arbiter of sex. In its absence, whether the constitution be XO, XX, XXX or even XXXX, the phenotype will be female. In its presence there will be a male—of sorts—even though the complement may be XXXXY.

In general (and there are always exceptions) sex chromosome anomalies do not cause intersex states if all the body cells develop from one stem line: if the complement in all cells is the same. However, if there be mosaicism with one stem line, let us say, bearing a Y and the other not, there may be intersex states. As Overzier has said, "It would seem that the majority of intersexes have passed through a stage of mosaicism in their early development". Note here the implication that stem lines can die out and that the final chromosome complement could be different from what it had been in the past.

The X Chromosome

As we have noted the two X chromosomes are those most nearly metacentric in group C. They are about the second in size of this rather indistinguishable array of pairs 6–12. How can we distinguish the X

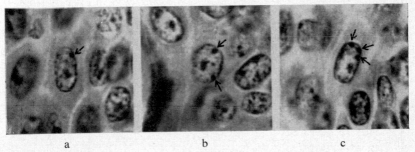

a   b   c

Fig. 68. Sex-chromatin Barr bodies. a: one Barr body, two X chromosomes, XX. b: two Barr bodies, three X chromosomes, XXX. c: three Barr bodies, XXXX. (*Preparation kindly supplied by Prof. Murray L. Barr*)

chromosome? How can we know if one is missing. How can we tell how many may be present in excess? Distinction can be made in more than one way.

When more than one X is present the other (or others) largely become inactive as they become condensed, hetero-pyknotic, their genetic ladder stacked. In this condensed condition they become visible as Barr bodies: tiny plano-convex masses about 1 μ in size lying against the inner surface of the nuclear membrane. If only one X is present its activities are fully required. It is extended and active. No Barr body is seen. If two are present, one Barr body will be seen; with three, two (Fig. 68). The number of X chromosomes is one more than the number of Barr bodies to be found (Fig. 69). One must state here that, possibly for technical reasons, not all cells examined will demonstrate this n minus 1 rule. Vaginal smears give a better correlation than buccal mucosal smears where, depending on the age of the subject and drugs which my be taken, the rule may be shown by between 25 and 50 per cent of cells. Sometimes two cell populations can be distinguished; if this be so one must suspect mosaicism. If there is a constant discrepancy between mucosal smears and karyotype, mosaicism should likewise be

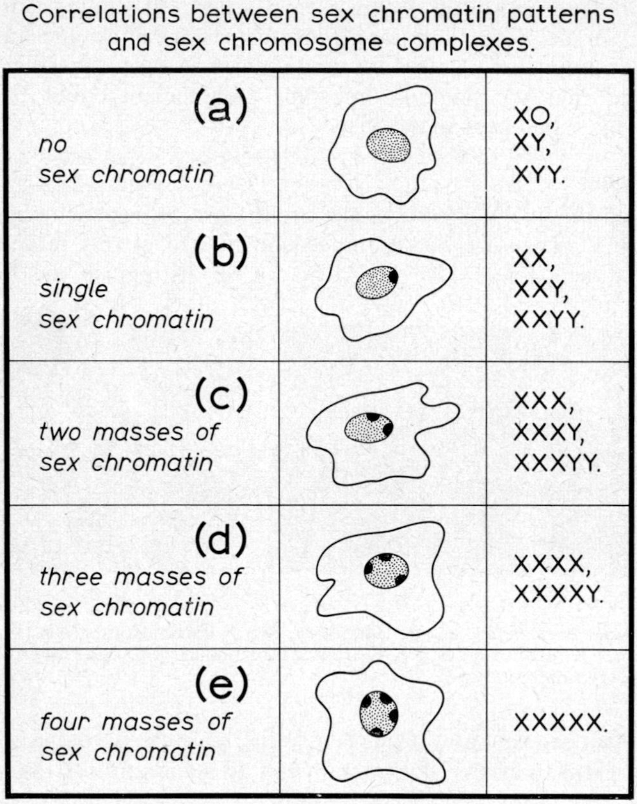

Correlations between sex chromatin patterns
and sex chromosome complexes.

(a) no sex chromatin		XO, XY, XYY.
(b) single sex chromatin		XX, XXY, XXYY.
(c) two masses of sex chromatin		XXX, XXXY, XXXYY.
(d) three masses of sex chromatin		XXXX, XXXXY.
(e) four masses of sex chromatin		XXXXX.

Fig. 69. Correlations between sex chromatin patterns and sex chromosome complements. (*From a drawing kindly supplied by Prof. M. L. Barr*)

suspected. It is a wise plan to do smears from both sides of the mouth and both lateral vaginal walls in cases with intersex features. I know of one case of mosaicism where the right side of the body was predominantly XX, the left side XO!

The "Drumsticks" of the polymorphs (Fig. 6) also give an indication of the number of X chromosomes but the n minus 1 rule for the number of drumsticks does not hold good to any reliable degree when more than two X chromosomes are present. One rarely sees two drumsticks with XXX; with XXXX one never sees three.

The X chromosome can be identified by autoradiography (Fig. 12) as a late-replicating large chromosome of the characteristics of a nearly metacentric C. That is to say it takes up more H_3-marked thymidine because it has not already partly taken up unmarked thymidine by partial replication before the H_3-thymidine was added.

The Lyon Hypothesis

The theory states, as we have said, that where one or more X chromosomes are present there is random inactivation of all except one in all the cells of the developing foetus at about the time of implantation. If there are two XX chromosomes, one is patroclinous (derived from father) and one matroclinous (maternally derived). In about half the cells one type will remain active while the other becomes condensed; in a complementary number of cells the other X will be the active one. Which chromosome is active in which cell seems to be a chance selection, but once the decision has been made descendants of all cells will perpetuate that chance selection for activity. One says "selection for activity" because cell activity is dependent on its genes, and may thus be dependent on which chromosome is active: matroclinous or patroclinous.

If a female zygote is heterozygous for an X-linked and detectable mutant gene (carries a normal gene on one X chromosome but an abnormal and detectable gene on the other), we may be able to detect that two cell populations in equal, or nearly equal, numbers, of different genetic quality, make up the body. Where the gene for the enzyme glucose-6-phosphate dehydrogenase is carried on one X, but not on the other, two red cell populations can be detected: one active for the enzyme, the other not. In X-linked muscular dystrophy, normal and abnormal muscle cells can be seen in the female heterozygous for that condition. In the newly described disease of X-linked Lisch-Nyham hyperuricacidaemia, where the enzyme hypoxanthine-guanine-phosphoribosyl transferase gene is missing from one X in the heterozygote carrier females of that condition, two cell populations can be found: those with normal metabolism of uric acid and those without.

Of course, where two X chromosomes are present, one cannot entirely be inactive. If it were thus, the normal XX individual would be phenotypically identical with she who is XO; and she is not. Likewise the XXX female would be the same as both those others, which often she is not. Clearly inactivation of the X in excess of one is partial only. There are said to be zones or gradations of inactivity.

The Y Chromosome

Although very similar in size and shape to the G group chromosomes, 21 and 22, it is not quite the same. It is a little bigger, the long arms tend to be closer together and, by H_3-thymidine labelling, it is later in replicating than 21 and 22.

Considerable variations in size are known to occur as normal and hereditary variants. In some normal persons the Y is much larger than is usual without detectable effect on phenotype. On the other hand partial deletions of Y have been reported in hypogonadism and inter-sexuality.

Of late much, indeed enormous, interest has centered on what, in addition to sex determination, the activities of the Y chromosome may be. In the last two years an avalanche of speculation and information has poured into the literature. In the past, apart from testis evocation in the foetus, it had been believed that the Y chromosome was perhaps concerned only with the triviality of a gene for a variety of hairy ears. Let us leave the new knowledge of the Y chromosome to Chapter XI. Let us say here only this: it seems more than likely that the Y chromosome shares some activities, is homologous with, the short arms of the X chromosome. At least, it seems to be so in some animals. In man it is less certain.

Some have debated whether X-bearing sperms can be distinguished from those that bear a Y. Is there perhaps "dimorphism". It now seems that perhaps they can be distinguished by phase contrast microscopy. If this be true, something at variance with our present beliefs has to be explained. From 20 young men, sperms were Y-bearing or X-bearing, not in a ratio of 1 : 1, but in a proportion of 168 : 100 respectively. If each sperm had as good a chance for fertilization as the other, the expected sex ratio of zygotes at conception would be the same: 168 : 100. One calculation of human sex ratio at conception has given just such a figure. Our ideas about sperm gametogenesis may have to be revised.

Mosaicism

Mosaics of sex chromosome anomalies are not uncommon; more common by far than, let us say, mongol mosaics. The reason may well be that sex chromosome anomalies, even the monosomy XO, are not so very lethal to the stem lines from which the mosaic individual develops. If non-disjunction of chromosome 21 occurs at the first mito-tic division of the zygote, two stem lines would be produced: one tri-somic 21, the other monosomic. Autosomal monosomies are always lethal, and the monosomic line would perhaps be expected to die out. The embryo would develop from the viable trisomic line. Perhaps many more mongols might have been mosaics but for this lethal effect.

If different stem lines of sex chromosome anomalies are formed they might be expected to survive and be perpetuated. This may be the reason why we see many and varied sex chromosome mosaics, XO/XX/XXX, XY/XO/XX, XY/XXY, XO/XY/XXY, XO/XY, XXXY/XXXXY, to name but a few of those that have been found.

It is in the study of the suspect mosaic that one must use all resources of investigation. Barr bodies may be sought in cells from several sites, drumsticks must be sought and counted. The study of Barr bodies and drumsticks, however, has its limitations, for both XO and XY cells will be chromatin negative; and XX cells and XXY cells will be positive. Tissue cultures may be made from more than one tissue: skin fibroblasts, bone marrow and from peripheral blood leucocytes. Autoradiographic studies with tritiated thymidine may also be required before one can be even reasonably sure just what stem lines are present.

Chapter X
Chromosome Anomalies in the Female

Gonadal Dysgenesis

The history of our knowledge of such disorders dates back to 1761 when Morgagni first described a case of congenital ovarian deficiency, but it is only in quite recent times that any great progress has been made in our understanding of gonadal dysgenesis.

It seems that it is better to use the term gonadal dysgenesis rather than gonadal aplasia for ovarian tissue is not entirely absent. The medullary portion of the ovary is present and rete tissue, hilus cells and stroma are to be found. It is germ cells that are lacking, and even they are not invariably entirely absent. There is some reason, as we have mentioned previously, to believe that in many cases germ cells may be present at an early stage of embryonic development, only to degenerate and disappear to greater or less degree as time goes on.

It seems that gonadal dysgenesis can be either genetically determined, and therefore potentially present from the beginning, or it may be acquired in the course of embryonic development.

The best known and most common variety is that in which, by deletion of either an X from an XX zygote or a Y from an XY zygote, the chromosome constitution is XO. There are variants of this variety depending on whether there is complete deletion, whether there may be deletion of the short arms only of the X chromosome (giving X$\bar{x}$), deletion of the long arms (giving X$\underline{x}$) or loss of either long or short arms by formation, respectively, of an isochromosome of the short arms or of the long arms of X giving X iso $\underline{x}$ or X iso $\bar{x}$ (see Fig. 16A, B). Deletions of an X chromosome, in whole or in part (and predominantly in whole) comprise the bulk of gonadal dysgenesis.

But chromosomal anomaly is not the only cause of failure of gonadal development. We are all familar with failure of an organ to develop for reasons which, while admittedly unknown, are not related to chromosome defect; we see sometimes renal agenesis, agenesis of a lung, anophthalmos. It is not a far cry to imagine that occasionally ovaries can fail to develop as the result of damage by vascular accident, viral influence or other causes. We can imagine, then, a female foetus, XX, suffering ovarian dysgenesis as a sole defect: "Pure gonadal dysgenesis".

If we have an XY male zygote who, for other than genetic and chromosomal reasons, has suffered failure of testis development at an early stage of embryonic growth we have a situation comparable to the rabbit embryos castrated in Jost's classic experiments. The phenotype develops along female lines. There is no gonad. So we have a female phenotype, an XY constitution and no gonads: Again "Pure Gonadal

126

Dysgenesis" but this time in an XY female (within our terms of reference.)

Turner's Syndrome, XO

Undoubtedly the best known variety of gonadal dysgenesis is that most usually called Turner's syndrome: The condition where failure of germ cell maturation is combined with short stature and an XO constitution. Sometimes a distinction is made wherein ovarian failure, short stature and an XO constituion is called the Bonnevie-Ullrich-Turner syndrome if certain other deformities are present. Webbing of the neck, cardio-vascular anomalies, telangiectasia, cubitus valgus and other defects are considered by some to put the patient into this separate category. There is some reason to believe that the presence or otherwise of these somatic deformities depends on how much of what part of the X chromosome is missing.

In the complete monosomy, XO, both long and short arms are missing. We then get gonadal dysgenesis, short stature and the multiple somatic stigmata of the Bonnevie-Ullrich-Turner syndrome. If the short arms only are missing we will get gonadal dysgenesis, short stature, and the stmigata of the Bonnevie-Ullrich-Turner syndrome. Genes for ovarian development, normal growth and negating the somatic stigmata seem to reside in the short arms of X. To simplify matters we can say that the constitution XO and X$\overline{\text{X}}$ give a short female with ovarian dysgenesis and what we will for brevity call Turner's syndrome·

If the long arms of one X are missing, X$\underline{\text{x}}$, we will get ovarian dys-genesis, because both arms seem necessary for gonad maturation, but we will not get short stature or the somatic stigmata.

While Turner's syndrome is not ordinarily a familial disease, more than one family has been reported where two sibs are affected. Whether this event represents an especial liability to abnormal chromosome segregation in the parents, or whether it is mere coincidence, we do not know. We do however now know from the work of Carr that those living cases of Turner's syndrome that we see are but a small residue of those that are conceived. Perhaps 98 per cent of XO conceptuses are rejected as miscarriages; only 2 per cent develop and are born alive. Whereas 5 per cent of aborted foetuses are XO, the incidence of Turner's syndrome is no more than about one in 2500 babies born.

The condition is not easy to diagnose in early infancy. It is true that in the three cases detected in the newborn survey of Maclean abnormalities could be discovered, but one suspects that those abnormalities were noted only after the abnormal chromosome constitution was known. However, there are features that might be recognized by an astute clinician.

The Turner syndrome baby is usually small. One-third are under 2500 grams at birth. There is a soft pitting lymphoedema of the hands and feet which persists for a few weeks or months. The hair-line at the neck is low, and even if no true webbing of the neck is present, the skin tends to be loose and redundant so that the baby might be picked up as a mother cat carries her kittens (Fig. 70). Even in early infancy it may be noted that the nipples are placed widely apart, and that the chest is broad and "shield-like".

Congenital cardio-vascular anomalies are common in this syndrome, and coarctation of the aorta—an extremely uncommon condition in

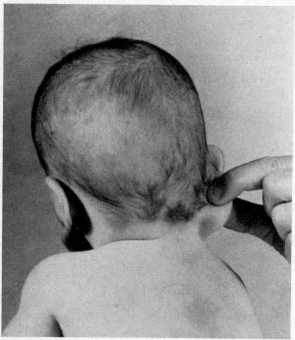

Fig. 70. Turner's Syndrome, baby Laura B. Although there is no true webbing of the neck, the skin of the neck is loose and redundant.

females without Turner's syndrome—is found in about one-quarter of the cases. Where the diagnosis is suspected, the femoral pulses should be sought. Coarctation of peripheral pulmonary arteries also may be present. It may happen that this or some other and more obvious cardiac deformity, pulmonary stenosis, ventricular septal defect, or patent ductus arteriosus, may call especial attention to a baby, whereupon close scrutiny will reveal to the clinician that the baby has Turner's syndrome.

Laura B. was referred at seven days of age for respiratory difficulty that was found to be due to cardiac failure. The femoral pulses could not be felt. The blood pressure in the arms was 160 mm. Hg. systolic; in the legs it was 60. No cardiac murmur was present at this time, but a diagnosis of coarctation of the aorta seemed likely. Because of the rarity of coarctation in normal females, the baby was examined closely, and there was found looseness of the skin illustrated in Fig. 70. Buccal mucosal smear showed no Barr body in any cells. The baby was chromatin negative and clearly XO. Angiography demonstrated the coarctation. A murmur appeared in a few weeks.

One must admit that had it not been for the cardiac failure due to the coarctation this case would have been missed and the baby would have been passed without qualification as suitable for adoption—as was the

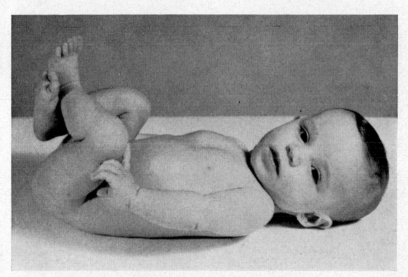

Fig. 71. Turner's Syndrome, baby Laura B. The diagnosis in infancy can be very difficult. This baby looks normal and would have escaped recognition had she not had coarctation of the aorta.

intent here. The diagnosis of the baby with Turner's syndrome is not easy. (Fig. 71). Many cases pass unrecognized in early life.

Even in later childhood the diagnosis is not obvious. The lymph-oedema disappears, the broad chest may not excite comment and the loose folds of skin may pass unnoticed unless a distinctive web is formed. However, shortness of stature is universal and should arouse suspicion. Any female who for no obvious reason of systemic disease or malnutrition is below the third percentile of normal height for her age (or two standard deviations below normal) must be considered as a possible case of Turner's syndrome and should be examined for other stigmata and by buccal smear.

In addition to the redundant loose skin about the neck, a true webbing (Fig. 72a), or mere flattening of the posterior contour of the neck with a

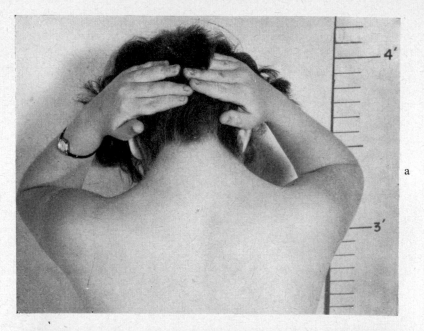

a

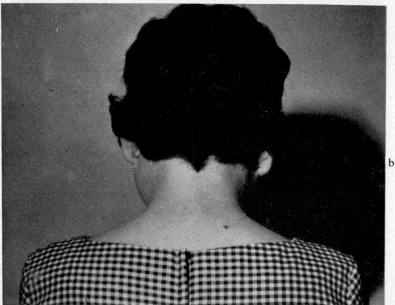

b

Fig. 72. Turner's Syndrome. a: Back view of girl on left of Fig. 73 showing webbed neck. b: The neck may scarcely appear abnormal, but a wide flat contour is usual. (*Photographs by courtesy of Dr Earl Plunkett*)

low hair-line, the shield-like chest should be sought. Cubitus valgus, an increased "carrying angle" at the elbow should be looked for, though this is not a very distinctive sign. The heart should be examined carefully for evidence of congenital defect, and the blood pressures in arms and legs estimated. Other features are often present in this syndrome. There is commonly a high arched palate, a receding chin and dental malocclusion. There may be bony defects of many kinds, though some deformity of the metacarpals is the most usual. General osteoporosis is often seen in an X-ray film. A pyelogram will very commonly reveal some anomaly of the urinary tract, and horseshoe kidney is not rare. Telangiectasias of the skin are sometimes found and telangiectasia of the bowel is an important, if somewhat rare, event. Deeply pigmented nevi are very common on the trunk and neck (Fig. 72b). Severe melaena and unexplained blood loss in a dwarfed girl might suggest the possibility of Turner's syndrome, especially since that other cause of symptomless severe melaena—a Meckel's diverticulum—is a rarity in girls. Finally one should remember that healing of wounds with keloid scarring is common in this syndrome: a matter of importance if plastic surgical correction of a webbed neck is contemplated.

The dermal ridge patterns are unusual. As has been indicated in our chapter on dermatoglyphics the patterns tend to be large and the total digital ridge count tends to be high. There is an increased frequency of large ulnar loops on the thumbs. Radial loops are less common on the second digit than might be expected; they are likely to be replaced by ulnar loops. The axis triradius, is often distal: in 50 per cent of cases of Turner's Syndrome against 10 per cent of normals. True patterns on the hypothenar eminences are thus not rare. A transverse palmar crease is more common than in normal females and a single fifth digit crease, almost unknown in normals, is sometimes seen. The hallucal patterns are very large; usually they are large distal loops or whorls with many ridges between core and triradii.

One does not expect to see or find all of these features in every case, but in gonadal dysgenesis of XO type, short stature is universal. An inexplicably short girl deserves a buccal mucosal smear.

Very often it is only when expected puberty fails to appear that there is real suspicion that something is truly amiss. The breasts fail to develop, pubic and axillary hair is absent or very sparse and menstruation does not occur (Fig. 73). The external genitalia are infantile and the vaginal lining is thin. Smears show no evidence of oestrogen activity. The body of the uterus is small, though the cervix is often of fair size. The tubes are thin and the mucosal folds dystrophic. The ovaries are represented by white streaks or knobs of largely fibrous tissue in which may be found remnants of rete tissue and mesonephros. Sterility, of course, is a virtual certainty though one case is reported to have borne a child.

That all this, and the short stature, is not due to pituitary failure is

C.D.   K certain, for there are normal levels of adrenotrophic and thyrotropic hormones. The pituitary gonadotrophic hormones are, indeed, much increased. It is as though the pituitary were trying to whip into activity a flagging gonad. In fact no such gonad exists in normal form. As a consequence of this increased gonadotrophic activity some degree of hypertension is quite common, and "hot flushes" may be experienced.

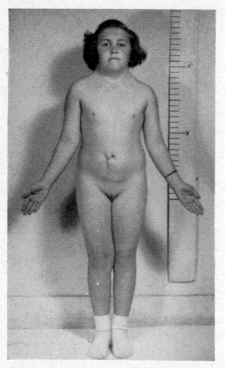 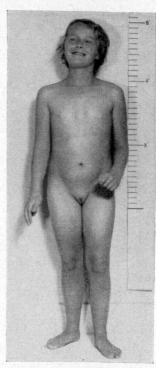

Fig. 73. Turner's Syndrome in Adolescence. The girl on the left with the webbed neck is fourteen years old, and that on the right nineteen. Note the short statures. Photographs taken before treatment. (*By courtesy of Dr Earl Plunkett*)

The outlook for mental development is a little uncertain. It does seem that appreciable mental retardation is unusual. These patients, it is true, tend to be timid, to lack ambition, and to be easily influenced by others, but the mean I.Q. of 20 cases was estimated at 98. Lack of libido and frigidity are common. It has been said that these patients suffer from "space form blindness", an impairment of judgement of spatial configurations.

Recently it has been shown that there appears to be a relationship between thyroid function and the chromosome disorders in general. In Turner's syndrome, while the protein-bound iodine levels are not unusual, the uptake by the thyroid gland of radioactive iodine, I^{131}, is above normal. Moreover, auto-antibodies against the thyroid gland are more commonly to be found in patients with Turner's syndrome, and in their normal-seeming relatives, than is to be expected. It has been suggested that a tendency to produce such antibodies may in some way be linked with abnormalities of chromosome segration.

Cytogenetic Features of Turner's Syndrome

In 80 per cent of cases of Turner's syndrome the constitution is 44 plus XO: Complete deletion of a sex chromosome, monosomy X. This is, with the exception of the unique case of monosomy 21, the only monosomy in mammals compatible with life; even YO is lethal. We are not sure from where the chromosome is lost. Is Y lost to a Y-bearing sperm; is X lost from an X sperm? Is the X in the XO Turner's syndrome always derived from mother (matroclinous), or may it be that the X is

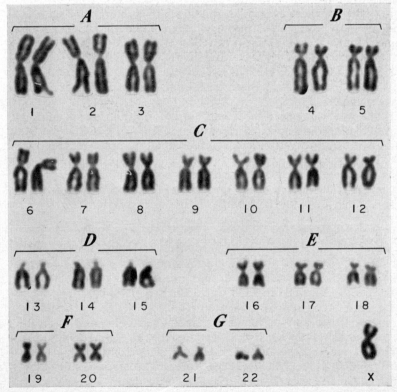

Fig. 74. Karyotype of XO Gonadal Dysgenesis with Turner's Syndrome. This is the commonest type of Gonadal Dysgenesis. (*Preparation by Dr D. H. Carr*)

missing from the female gamete and that the X comes from the father? We are not sure.

It does not seem very likely that the loss is by non-disjunction at meiosis in the mother, for there is no age-dependent risk in Turner's syndrome. On the other hand twin births are more common in an XO sibship than might be expected, and this surely suggest a maternal cause. On the other hand studies of colour-blindness, and of the Xg blood group system seem to show that in some cases the X is matroclinous and that it is the sperm that has been deleted of X or Y. However all that may be, in the great majority of Turner's syndrome cases the Karyotype is XO (Fig. 74).

As we have indicated, there may be variants showing gonadal dysgenesis with great or less degree of other stigmata. Some are examples of mosaicism, XX/XO. Some with short stature only and perhaps less degree of somatic stigmata will show short arm deletion $X\bar{x}$; or they may show isochromosome of the long arms (that is to say, have long arms only) and be X iso-$\bar{x}$.

In "pure" gonadal dysgenesis, one third of cases are apparently XX, and one must presume that primary ovarian failure has come about by some early embryonic accident not of chromosomal cause. Two-thirds are apparently XY. One says "apparently" because they may not be truly XY at all. It could be that they really are X$\underline{x}$ and that the apparent Y is really the remaining short arms of X. The appearances could be quite similar.

In the event that one of the X chromosomes is abnormal it seems that nature reduces the degree of defect in an ingenious, if mysterious, way. The abnormal chromosomes seem preferentially to be selected for partial inactivation at the "time of decision" in the embryo. If there is partial deletion of one X, let us say X$\underline{x}$, the Barr body will be unusually small. If there is reduplication of the long arms to make a bigger-than-usual chromosome, iso-$\bar{x}$, the Barr body will be larger than normal.

"Turner's Syndrome" in Males

Occasionally males are seen with short stature, webbed necks, congenital heart disease, and other stigmata that are described as somatic manifestations of Turner's syndrome, but one has to remember that what Turner described in 1938 was a phenotypic picture. He did not define the aetiology. There may be other causes of Turner's constellation of stigmata than an X chromosome anomaly. In the same way that all bleeding diseases are not due to haemophilia, all stigmata of Turner's syndrome may not be due to X deletion. The Turner phenotype has been reported as recurring from generation to generation of one family. Affected females were fertile and had offspring, males and females, XY and XX who showed the stigmata apparently determined by an X-linked dominant gene.

One could invoke chromosome disorder in these male cases by postulating mosaicism. Indeed one case has been so explained. He seemed to have the complex constitution, X, iso-$\bar{x}$/X, iso-$\bar{x}$/iso-Y. Mosaicism is to the cytogeneticist as are "variable expression" and "diminished penetrance" to the geneticist; a fine way out of trouble.

But the male with stigmata of Turner's syndrome could arise in yet another way. If we assume, as some have done, that the short arms of X and short arms of Y have certain genes in common (that there are homologous segments) we could presume that the relevant segments, those that negate certain stigmata, are lost from the Y chromosome of the male Turner's syndrome case; but their loss is undetectable.

Clinical Management of Gonadal Dysgenesis and Turner's Syndrome

It is repeating a platitude to state that one must not only treat the disease but that one must also manage and help the patient. One must be most mindful of this in sex chromosome anomalies. Sexual function is matter charged with great emotional content for the patient. One must not mention under any circumstances that the patient is "only half a woman" or "half-way towards a man". She is not. She is a woman whose puberty has not yet taken place. The reader may agree with me that chromosomes are hard enough for us to understand! How can a patient comprehend them? Cytogenetic explanations are best avoided. If the diagnosis seems certain on the basis of primary failure of ovarian function, a high gonadotrophin level, short stature and a chromatin negative buccal mucosal smear, one need go little further, though one would look carefully for coarctation of the aorta and renal tract anomalies. Laparotomy or culdoscopy are not essential to the diagnosis of Turner's syndrome.

One must then explain, perhaps with a half-truth, that the ovaries are not putting out the hormone required to bring on puberty, breast development and menstruation. One can draw an analogy between her disease and the failure of the pancreas to put out insulin in diabetes. This she will likely understand. One would not rush to tell an adolescent that she will never have a baby of her own. The time for that is some way off. At any age a patient may be much distressed by such news, and teenage girls are especially sensitive in such things.

The time will come, however, when the subject must be discussed. In an older woman (or in a young one if marriage is even on the horizon) one must tell the truth: that you can offer her everything except fertility. It must now be explained that, not only does the ovary not make hormones, but that it does not make egg-cells. This cannot be put right. One must make sure that she understands that her disease, if treated, is no barrier to full sex satisfaction for both parties, and that she will not be frigid and unresponsive. This is important. It is, of course, only fair and right that an intended spouse should be informed of her inability to bear a baby of her own. Your patient may wish to do this for herself, or may wish to bring her fiance to talk with you. In either event, such words as "infertility" and "sterility" are best avoided. An "inability to bear a baby of her own" will suffice. Needless to say, one will point out that many happy couples are in the same position, and that adoption will give them joy and satisfaction.

The pharmacological management of the ovarian failures is the replacement of the oestrogen deficiency that has made them appear different from their fellows, irrespective of their karyotypes. Society is not concerned with chromosomes. It is concerned with toilet habits and with sexual role. These patients will go to the "Ladies". It behoves us, then, to make them as near to ladies as we can. Cyclic oestrogen therapy is used in Turner's syndrome and in the "pure" gonadal dysgenesis.

Stilboestrol is satisfactory. For the first year or so 2 mgm. daily may be given for three weeks, stopped for a week and recommenced for a further three weeks. A larger dose, perhaps 5 mgm. daily, may be used after a few months if nausea is not a problem. A progestogen may be given in addition more closely to mimic a normal period. Under this treatment the breasts will develop and a normal feminine figure will appear, though it may take several months for full maturation. Development of internal and external genitalia will improve their ability for normal sexual intercourse, and there will be improvement in libido. Psychological maturation will also occur, and a young girl previously dull and reticent may become more self-confident, modest, but flirtatious. Such are the benefits of oestrogens.

Unfortunately, growth of these short women does not occur with treatment. Indeed one might be worried that too early treatment of a girl approaching the age of natural puberty would result in a too early closure of the epiphyses and even greater stunting. One should perhaps wait until 14 years of age, though one must be aware that so to delay pubescence might be a distressing embarrassment to a girl surrounded by her blossoming peers.

Testicular Feminization Syndrome, XY

This is an intersex state characterized by female internal genitalia, normal breasts, no uterus, yet testes and the chromosome complement XY.

This appears to be an hereditary disorder inherited either as a sex-linked recessive trait or possibly as a sex-limited autosomal dominant. In the former case the mutant gene would be carried on one X chromosome with a normal allele on the other X. An XY zygote, hemizygous for the X bearing the abnormal gene, and having therefore no normal allele, would exhibit the effect of the abnormal gene. If the disorder were to be carried as a sex-limited autosomal dominant characteristic the situation would be that both XX and XY zygotes would equally be at risk (as an even chance) of receiving the abnormal gene, but that its effect, like baldness for example, would be exhibited only by an individual with an XY constitution.

In the last year or two, whatever the method of genetic transmission may be, the manner of causation of the syndrome seems to have become clear. There is unresponsiveness of the primordial genitalia to the androgenic steroid produced by the embryonic testis.

As the result of the XY constitution the medullary portion of the primitive gonad is stimulated; a testis forms. Let there be no mistake, the gonads are testes. These testes produce an androgenic steroid, as does the normal foetal testis. This steroid does not appear to be abnormal; but the tissue reaction to it is. There is no response, no male development, no penis, no scrotum, only a continuation of development on female lines: a female phenotype. We have then an XY child, to all external appearances a girl. The testes do not descend fully and remain within the abdomen, or at best within the inguinal canal.

As time goes on, and the patient reaches the age of puberty, gonadophic hormones stimulate these testes. They respond by output of androgenic hormones and, as is normal in the normal testis, some oestrogenic steroids also. The tissues cannot, and do not, respond to the androgenic steroids from the testis; there is no growth of beard or male pubic hair, no growth of phallus and no deepening of voice. The pituitary fails to "recognize" the androgen and, in an effort to call to life what seems to it to be an idle gonad, produces greater quantities of gonadotrophic hormones. The testis responds and makes more androgen and oestrogen. Only the oestrogen evokes a body response. The body configuration is female, voluptuous breasts develop. Our patient becomes beautiful and sumptuously endowed but is, for all that, equipped with testes and an XY complement. These patients, I am told, are to be found among the ranks of show-girls. Regretably we have no illustration of an adult patient for our book!

The testes of these patients are not normal. The seminferous tubules are immature, and the lining epithelium is formed of layers of undifferentiated and abnormal Steroli cells. Germ cells are rarely seen. The interstitial cells, by contrast, are well developed and may show adenomatous proliferation. Often the testes are ectopic: 60 per cent are in the inguinal canal, 20 per cent in the labia majora and 20 per cent remain in the abdomen.

In infancy and childhood no abnormality is likely to be noted, but where an inguinal hernia is found in a female child we must bear in mind that a gonad at that site may be, not a prolapsed ovary, but a testis. Remember the testicular feminization syndrome (Fig. 75).

When the expected time of puberty falls due it will become apparent that all is not well. While breasts will develop ample proportions, there

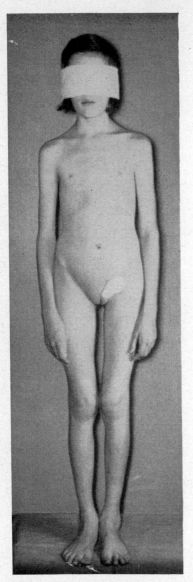

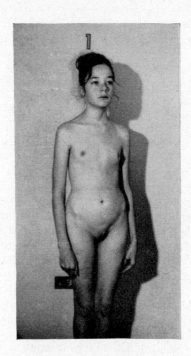

Fig. 75. Testicular Feminization Syndrome. On the left, at age twelve, she was found to have bilateral inguinal masses, at first thought to be hydrocoeles of the Canal of Nuck. They were found to be testes and were removed. There is no uterus, and the vagina is about two inches long. On the right she is aged fourteen and has been taking œstrogens for eighteen months. Breasts are developing and there is some growth of pubic hair. (*Case history and photographs kindly supplied by Dr F. Doerffer, Hamilton, Ontario*)

will be primary amenorrhoea. Pubic and axillary hair will be sparse or absent.

These women are unusually tall with an average height of five feet eight inches; some are nearly six feet. They are handsome and attractive, intelligent and often ambitious. Libido may be increased. The internal genitalia are infantile. The vagina may be quite short; in any event it will end blindly, for there is no uterus. Swellings, the ectopic testes, are likely to be found in the labia majora or the inguinal canals (Fig. 75).

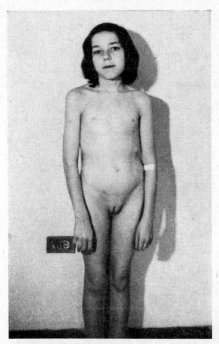

Fig. 76. Testicular Feminization Syndrome. This girl is the sister of Fig. 75. An inguinal hernia was repaired as an infant and a testis found. At eight years of age she has not yet been started on œstrogen therapy. (*History and photograph kindly supplied by Dr F. Doerffer, Hamilton, Ontario*)

There seems to be debate as to how they may best be managed. Some, fearing malignant change, advocate removal of the abnormal testes followed by replacement oestrogen therapy. Others, stating that the risk of malignant change is no more than five per cent, are opposed to this castration for, they say, the abnormal testes are producing oestrogens—and this is what is wanted. Perhaps a compromise might be the best: that the testes are not removed until breast development is complete, that abdominal testes be removed for they cannot readily be observed, that inguinal and labial testes be closely observed for any change in size or consistency and that additional oestrogens be given, if external genital development is inadequate for normal sex relations. Vaginoplasty may be needed.

It goes without saying that the patient must not be told that she is anything but a woman. The fact that she has testes must be a closely guarded secret. Television and magazine expositions of biology have made the public quite sophisticated. Many people know that "XY" means "male". Mention of chromosomes is best avoided. She may be told that the womb has not developed normally, that the sex-glands are not working as they should and that she will be unable to have children of her own. Provided the vagina is adequate there will be no obstacle to normal sex relations. Some of her "sisters" may have the same disorder (Fig. 76). Female sibs should have their chromosomes examined.

Polysomy of X: Triple-, Tetra-, and Penta-X (XXX, XXXX, and XXXXX)

In these disorders, by non-disjunction at either the first meiotic division, at the second, or at both (Fig. 20) two, three, or four X chromosomes are present in a gamete. Fertilization adds another. It is believed that it is

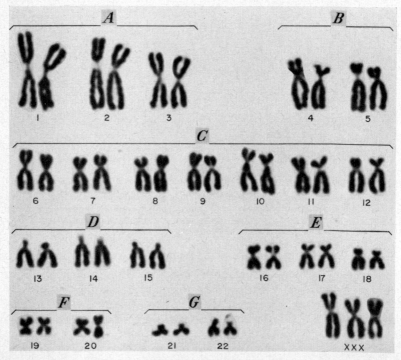

Fig. 77. Karyotype of female, XXX. The term "super-female" has now been discarded and the term "Triple-X" is used. (*Preparation by Dr D. H. Carr*)

more usually the maternal gamete that is at fault though the relation of the multiple X syndromes to maternal age is much less clear, if demonstrable at all, than in the syndromes involving autosome excesses. Errors of paternal gametogenesis, with a sperm bearing extra X's are quite within the bounds of possibility.

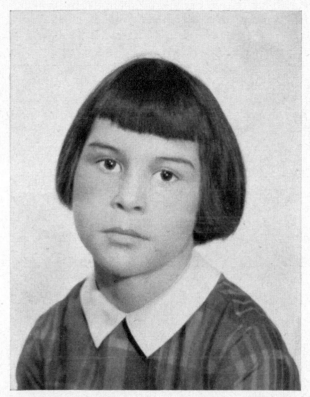

Fig. 78. Janet M, aged eight years, Triple-X, XXX. Her appearance is entirely normal. She is slightly retarded with an I.Q. of about 75. She was found on routine screening of retarded children. Pubertal development and reproductive function will be normal. Not all are retarded, and there may be many such amongst us. (*By kind permission of Dr G. Hinton*)

These patients are, as we would expect, chromatin positive on a buccal mucosal smear. They are chromatin-two (Fig. 68b), chromatin-three (Fig. 68c) and chromatin four positive, depending on whether the complement is XXX, XXXX or XXXXX. The n minus one rule holds good.

Although of more frequent occurrence than Turner's syndrome, in a ratio of three to one, the XXX female is likely to pass unrecognized, for in general, she shows no abnormality except on a buccal smear or karyotype (Fig. 77). She is a phenotypically normal female with normal pubescence, ovulation and fertility. Cases have in fact been found by chance. Even the dermal ridge patterns are not unusual though ridge counts on the digits may be low. The term "super-female" has no validity and has been abandoned.

One might expect that her offspring would be abnormal by secondary non-disjunction (Fig. 19) and that she would produce children in a

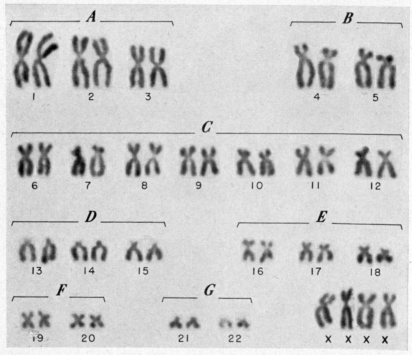

Fig. 79. Karyotype of Tetra-X female, XXXX. She was mentally retarded. (*Preparation by Dr D. H. Carr*)

ratio thus: two normals (XX or XY), one XXX and one XXY. Such, oddly, is not the case. There seems to be discrimination against abnormal conception and her children are all normal.

She may, however, have problems, for mental disturbance or psychotic behaviour is, perhaps, found in a greater number of Triple-X females than in the population as a whole (Fig. 78), but it is difficult to know if this is a valid observation for it is more among retarded patients in institutions that surveys have been made than among normal females. All we can say is this: in a large female newborn population the incidence was 0·12 per cent; in an institution for the retarded 0·5 per cent. In an institution for mentally disturbed females 11 of 22 **XXX** females had "normal I.Q's" but had psychiatric disorders, including schizophrenia.

Tetra-X(**XXXX**) (Fig. 79) patients are rare and invariably retarded. Within the last month the author has seen a penta-X (**XXXXX**) girl. She was grossly retarded, of small stature and immature sexual development, her features were coarse and prognathic but no other definite abnormality was found.

Chapter XI
Sex Chromosome Anomalies in Males

Klinefelter's Syndrome

In 1942, Klinefelter and his associates described a syndrome of asperma-togenesis and gynaecomastia in males. The name "Klinefelter's Syndrome" is in general use, though "Testicular Dysgenesis" and "Chromatin Positive Micro-orchidism" have also been proposed. In 1956 Bradbury and his co-workers and Plunkett and Barr, showed that these patients were chromatin positive, suggesting the presence of two X chromosomes. In 1959 Jacobs and Strong showed that there were indeed two X chromosomes. The karyotype in the most usual variety of this syndrome is XXY. This has amply been confirmed.

The incidence of this disorder and its chromosomal variants is about one in every 500 males according to the latest information. In a study of 663 boys in a school for the mentally handicapped a much higher incidence was found: 12 per 1000.

The disorder can scarcely be detected in infancy and childhood. Even knowing that the condition existed in their patients, Maclean and his colleagues could find no clinically evident disorder in the newborn males; nor is any abnormality to be found on examination of the child before puberty, unless there be slight mental retardation.

When the time of puberty is reached there may be some delay in its appearance but this slight delay is neither constant nor striking. The body build may be slightly unusual in that the limbs tend to be long and the overall height somewhat greater than average. Many such patients are tall, thin, and of delicate girlish appearance, but some are sthenic, heavy, and plethoric (Fig. 80). Others again are entirely normal. In about 30 per cent, and especially in those that are of heavy build, the breasts are enlarged, mostly by deposits of fat. One or two cases of cancer of the breast in males have been in cases of this syndrome. The hands and feet are large.

The mentality may be entirely normal but more usually the patients are unambitious, dependent and submissive. Behavioural difficulties and delinquency are common. Overt mental retardation, though not of great degree, is found in some 25 per cent. The electroencephalogram is often abnormal. Although sexual drive and potency are often subnormal, some patients cover their defects by boasts of their prowess with the ladies.

The penis is usually of normal or only slightly small size. The pubic hair is sparse and usually of female distribution. The beard is often slow to develop and scanty. The voice may be somewhat feminine in pitch. While prior to puberty the testes are not discernably smaller than

144

average, after that time they are clearly abnormally small. They may be either soft or hard.

The changes in the testes seem to increase with puberty under the influence of the pituitary gonadotrophins which are always at a high level. There are no very striking histological changes before that time. The seminferous tubules become narrow or obliterated and hyaline

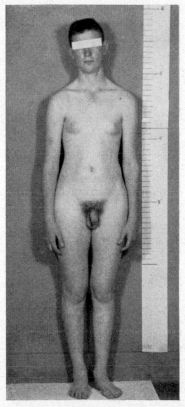
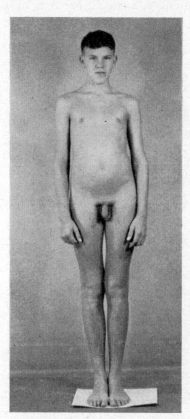

Fig. 80. Klinefelter's Syndrome, XXY. Note the different body builds, the female type of pubic escutcheon and the breast development in the left-hand figure. (*Kindly supplied by Dr Earl Plunkett*)

sclerosis is characteristic. Those tubules that are not sclerosed are lined by Sertoli cells, but these cells may be degenerate. Leydig's interstitial cells appear to be increased because the other elements of the testes are reduced in quantity. Spermatogenesis is usually entirely absent but in some tubules some spermatogenesis may be seen.

A reduced uptake of I^{131} by the thyroid gland gives evidence of disordered function. The dermal ridges may show slight departures from normal in that the axis triradii tend, if anything, to be in a more distal position than is usual; and the atd angle is somewhat increased. There are perhaps more arches on the digits than is normal, and the ridge count of loops tends to be low.

As one can see, apart from tiny testes in the adult, there are no constant clinical features of this syndrome. The chief problem of these patients is infertility. Some 40 per cent of aspermic males are examples of this syndrome.

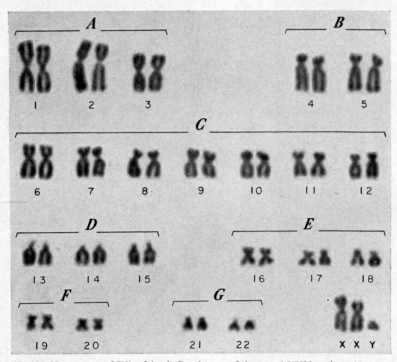

Fig. 81. Karyotype of Klinefelter's Syndrome of the usual XXY variety. (*Preparation by Dr D. H. Carr*)

Cytogenetic Features of Klinefelter's Syndrome

In the usual and much most common variety the karyotype is XXY: an extra X is present in this undoubted male (Fig. 81). The buccal mucosal smear will show a Barr body in the cell nuclei: there is an X chromosome in excess of one, and this will be condensed, heteropyknotic and visible (Fig. 68a). Just why this excess X should cause the changes that it does is far from clear.

Where does the extra X come from? There is a very slight, maybe significant, relation to maternal age, and thus it may be that a normal sperm brings a Y chromosome to a non-disjuncted XX ovum; or it may be that an XY-bearing sperm joins with a normal ovum. We cannot say.

It can happen, though rarely, that more than one X chromosome is present in excess. The karyotype will be XXXY (Fig. 82) and the buccal mucosal smear will be chromatin-two positive (Fig. 68b). A fault of segregation of the chromosomes at one level of gametogenesis in both parents might be postulated, but it is much more likely that non-

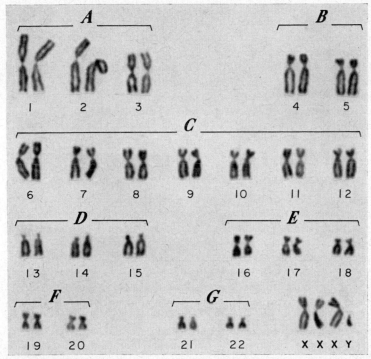

Fig. 82. Karyotype of XXXY variant of Klinefelter's Syndrome. (*Preparation by Dr D. H. Carr*)

disjunction at both meiotic divisions in one parent has taken place (Fig. 20). The XXY individual presents features little different from the regular Klinefelter's syndrome, XXY, except so far as mental function is concerned. All are mentally retarded.

As may be seen also from Fig. 20, four X chromosomes could be present in one gamete. If fertilization should add a Y, the "pentasomic" state XXXXY would result. An individual with this constitution has Klinefelter's syndrome, but with new features; a considerable number of cases have been reported. Severe mental defect is the rule, and of course infertility; but in addition there are special features: a large broad nose, large mouth and prognathos. Large ears are seen and maybe squints and epicanthic folds. Radio-ulnar synostosis is usual with restricted supination of the forearms. The joints tend otherwise to be hyperextensible and there is hypotonia and often scoliosis. There may be coxa valga and pes planus. The buccal smear is chromatin three positive (Fig. 68c).

Two other variants of Klinefelter's syndrome are known to occur. There are those patients who are XXYY, and one is reported who is XXXYY. The former patients are not different phenotypically from the regular Klinefelter's syndrome patients, XXY, save in one respect: The dermal ridge patterns are characteristic. There is a triradius to the ulnar side of the palm, an "ulnar triradius", and there are hypothenar patterns: loop carpal, loop radial or arch radial. Arches and very small loops are often found on the fingers. The one XXXYY patient with 49 chromosomes in all, apart from showing Klinefelter's syndrome changes in the testes and severe mental retardation, showed also gigantism and acromegaly.

The YY Complement

When I wrote on this subject four years ago I dismissed an excess of Y chromosomes in just a few lines. I am not sure, despite an enormous interest in the YY syndrome by many workers, that what I write now will add substantially to the truth of what I wrote in 1965: "The XYY State produces no very constant effects. It is true that mental retardation has been found in some males . . . . The association may be fortuitous only, and related to the selection of cases examined. Certainly the XYY male can be normal and fertile. We do not know how many such are in our midst." Since then a spate of writings upon this subject has flowed over the medical literature, into the lay press and glossy magazines. Physicians and priests, philosophers, and moralists, judges and juries, a perplexed public and perturbed parents have come to take an interest in the Y chromosome and in the significance of its double representation on an individual's karyotype. I will see what I can sift from this innundation of biological fact and forensic fantasy.

Although a man with the XYY complement had been discovered, if not by accident at least unexpectedly (when investigated because he had a mongol child) in 1961, no great interest was aroused until 1965. Because it had been realized by Court Brown that there was a propensity to delinquency in patients with sex chromosome anomalies, Casey and his colleagues investigated the inmates of the Rampton and Moss Side institutions in England. In these institutions are held mentally subnormal individuals with anti-social and psychopathic personality defects. They found that of 942 male patients, 21 were chromatin positive, indicating that two X chromosomes were present in these males. Of these 21 chromosomally abnormal men, 12 had the complement XXY (and were thus cases of regular Klinefelter's Syndrome) but seven had the constitution XXYY. They noted the "extraordinary excess of individuals with the XXYY chromosome complement" in this security institution.

Jacobs and her co-workers acting on this hint, and noting the discrepancy between Casey's findings and those of Maclean who found only two XXYY cases in 2607 mentally retarded psychopaths without anti-social behaviour, considered the possibility that the extra Y chromosome predisposed its carriers to unusually aggressive behaviour. In her initial investigation she found seven examples of the complement XYY among 197 male inmates of Carstairs Institution in Scotland: an incidence of 3·5 per cent. Along with these seven XYY males there was one which was XXYY. Continuation of her study revealed nine XYY cases in a total of 315 inmates tested. Since it was believed that the incidence of the XYY constitution was no more frequent than perhaps one in 1500 of a control population, these findings seemed highly significant. It certainly seemed as though the XYY constitution predisposed to mental subnormality with aggressive anti-social behaviour.

Jacobs also noted that those with the XYY complement were unusually tall, and Price and his colleagues, working with the same sample, noted that six of the nine XYY men were over 72 inches (181 cms.). Jacobs has remarked "in this particular group a man more than 72 inches in height has approximately a one in two chance of having an XYY constitution". It has also been said: "half of all men over six feet in special security institutions are XYY—probably an exaggeration, but unlikely to be a very gross one".

These facts seemed to indicate that an extra Y chromosome was indeed associated with both aggressive delinquency and unusual height, though Hunter makes the point that "it might be that because of their great height and build they would present such a frightening picture that the court and psychiatrists would be biased to direct them to special hospitals for community safety".

The question of height in relation to XYY remains a little uncertain. Hunter, selecting those over the 90th percentile for height from 1021 inmates of an "Approved School" for boys of 12–19 years, found that three out of 29 examined were XYY; surely a high incidence. On the other hand, Welch and his colleagues, selecting 92 inmates over 72 inches from 464 males in a Maryland institution for "defective delinquents", and again from these selecting 10 who had I.Q. tests below 75, found no example of XYY—and yet these were among the most aggressive inmates of the institution. They wondered if their low incidence of XYY might be explained by the fact that many of their subjects were Negroes and if there might be a racial difference in the incidence of XYY. It has however been reported in a Negro.

Whether seizures and electroencephalographic abnormalities are a

regular feature of those with the XYY complement also is in some
doubt. Certainly a number of cases have been reported to have an
abnormal E.E.G. Indeed Forssman goes as far as to suggest that "one
should consider the possibility of double Y chromosomes in strikingly
tall men with epilepsy".

What does all this mean? Does it mean that all those that are XYY
are destined to psychopathic behaviour, criminality and incarceration?
Certainly not, for we have already noted that the first case of XYY ever

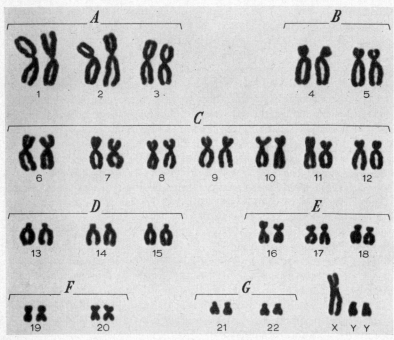

Fig. 83. XYY Karyotype. Although about one of every forty inmates of maximum
security institutions for the incorrigibly delinquent have this karyotype we have
found four examples in 1066 consecutive newborn males. The significance of this
karyotype is at present uncertain. (*Preparation by the Cytogenics Laboratory,
Victoria Hospital, London, Ontario*)

to be found was in a normal man. Is XYY, then, commonly, rarely or
only exceptionally associated with delinquent behaviour and conflict
with society? This question cannot be answered until we know how
many respectable and normal citizens, XYY, are in our midst. It cannot
be known until we have learned how many XYY babies are to be found
in a random population of newborns, and until we have followed those
we have found through infancy and childhood into adolescence and
maturity.

It has been estimated that the incidence of XYY may be between one in 1500 and one in 2000 males. Nobody really knows. We in this centre have reason to believe that the incidence may be much higher than previously has been thought. In 1066 consecutive newborn males born to mothers from all strata of society, Sergovich found four to be XYY (Fig. 83). In the same number he found one baby to be XXY.

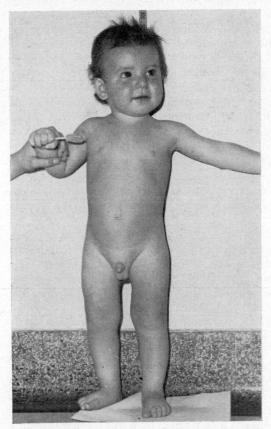

Fig. 84. XYY phenotype at age 15 months. Patient found at routine screening of consecutive newborns.

I have followed the oldest of these babies for only 20 months. Thus far all are entirely normal in growth, development and personality (Fig. 84). What does the future hold for them? Time alone will tell. Our newborn study shows that the ratio of XYY to XXY is roughly the same as that found in pooled data of security institutions: If this be so, we could deduce that the XYY anomaly was no more conducive to criminal insanity than is Klinefelter's syndrome. Perhaps the whole matter has been given too much attention by the press; perhaps scientists have been unwise in their prognostications. As Court Brown has said "It will be extremely important for doctors to control their enthusiasm and scientific pride, and prevent the non-expert from making exaggerated deductions."

I think we must grant, though, that the XYY complement gives some increased risk of anti-social, illegal behaviour. How does this show itself?

In the first place, as Price and Whatmore have shown, there is no family history of delinquent behaviour as there is so often in the case of criminality. The XYY delinquent is the "black sheep" of a law-abiding family. In infancy they may be entirely normal, but two of the three infants under my observation have exceeded the 97th percentile for body length. (But we do not know if they will have deviant behaviour.) One little boy, recently reported in the literature, started his mischief at two years of age. He often strayed away from home. Aged four-and-a-half he was destructive, defiant of authority, unmanageable. He kicked his baby brother and the cat, set fire to his room and was fearless in climbing ladders and window ledges. At five he took to sharp instruments and rammed a screwdriver into a small girl's abdomen. Aged eight he took to truancy and long distant wanderings. His intelligence was normal.

The picture in later life has been of irresponsibility, an unawareness of any but the immediate consequence of actions. There is inability to tolerate even mild frustrations. Few constructive ambitions or realistic goals are held. In general the criminal behaviour is directed more against property than persons, though there are grisly and notable exceptions. Arson especially seems to be a weakness.

Most of these men are of subnormal intellect, but few are severely retarded. Several are known to have an I.Q. of over 120; one is reported to rate as high as 135. All are, in comparison to their families, very tall, but all are not tall in relation to the population as a whole. Varicose ulcers of the legs are said to be common. Some have claimed that acne is more common in these patients. It has been claimed that in XYY adults the electrocardiogram is abnormal and shows a prolonged P–R interval (it is normally a little longer in XY men than XX women) and a secondary R wave and notching of S in the QRS complex of V_1. These were not found in two of our XYY infants.

Not too much seems to be known about their fertility. Undoubtedly they are not sterile; one patient has fathered seven children. Fertility may be reduced by lack of opportunity. Homosexuality has been reported.

There seems to be an increased output of testosterone. Pituitary follicle-stimulating hormone is reported as being normal, while leuteinizing hormone is much increased; the F.S.H. : L.H. ratio is perhaps

0·2 : 1 (normal 1–2 : 1). In spite of this, their genitalia appear quite normal and the testes are of normal size and consistency. Indeed there is nothing in body form, except stature, that singles out the XYY male. The testes have been stated on biopsy to show some features of Klinefelter's syndrome. This is hard to understand for it has also been reported that biopsy shows XY spermatocytes and there is reason to believe that fertility is not much, if at all, impaired. If they have children they are, so far as knowledge goes, of normal constitution. There seems to be selection against an XY or YY sperm though in theory their children could be XX, XY, XXY, or XYY. The fathers of two of my four XYY infants have normal karyotypes.

What of the moral and legal aspects of this disorder? This is a thorny question. As Dr. Elkinton has pertinently enquired: "Does the presence of such a genetic defect lessen the ethical and legal responsibility of an individual for his acts: If it does not mitigate his guilt, should it modify the nature of his sentence . . . . At what point does an anti-social person with abnormal chromosomes cease to be a criminal under the jurisdiction of the law and become a patient under the care of the medical profession. These are basic questions, but there are many more. If a newborn child is found to have an XYY pattern, what does one predict about his behaviour in later life? And what does one do about it?" (Fig. 85).

Let us take the last question first. I believe that in our present imperfect state of knowledge of its implications we should keep the discovery of the XYY chromosome constitution a secret, even from the parents—if one can. I can imagine no situation more likely to lead to abnormal upbringing of a child than for it to be known that the stage perhaps is set for a life of crime. The child must receive the benefit of the doubt. He is innocent until he acts otherwise.

It is not always possible to conceal this knowledge. It has so happened that two of my four babies were candidates for adoption. I felt it my duty to inform the adoption agency of our findings, with the recommendation that a frank exposition of our knowledge—and of our ignorance—be given to any prospective adopting parents. To act otherwise would be, I think, base deceit.

The father of one of the others, a high-school teacher, became curious at our interest in his normal baby, conceal it as we might. We explained that an "abnormality had been found in blood cells" but that (thinking of XXX) similar findings usually had no significance. He did some thinking and a week or two later asked "have you found a chromosome abnormality"? The answer had to be "yes". A few weeks passed. Our local press was full of the YY syndrome. He called again and asked "Is it an extra Y?" What could one say but, "yes".

Professor Trevor Gibbens, a leading authority on forensic psychiatry in Britain has written: "It seems to me doubtful whether evidence of

chromosome abnormality will give rise to any new issues in Court . . . .
If a man had no detectable abnormality except an XYY chromosome
constitution, it is very unlikely that this would be regarded in itself as
evidence of diminished responsibility." Here he speaks for the English
judicial system, but he continues: "In many foreign countries a particular crime must be punished by a particular sentence, unless the offender

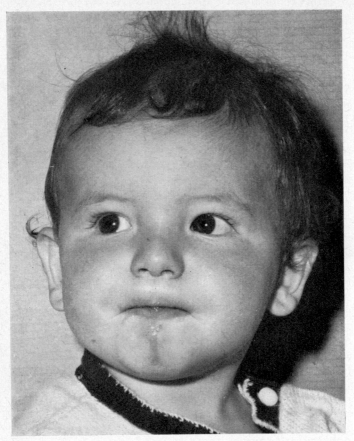

Fig. 85. David H: Phenotype XYY. What does the future hold? What should one
do about it?

is 'irresponsible'; so that it is vital to find evidence of irresponsibility.
. . . In England . . . the courts are free to take whatever social action is
necessary to protect society or provide remedial treatment of the
offender, whatever his state of 'responsibility'." Surely this is the
sensible approach. In this light the chromosomes, XYY or otherwise,
become irrelevant. In Melbourne, Australia, an XYY man was acquitted

of wilful murder. The jury took into account his genetic constitution. In France a jury decided that an XYY man was indeed responsible for his actions and convicted him of murder but with a light sentence. The tall, dull, acned and convicted slayer of eight Chicago student nurses is rumoured to be XYY. One awaits with interest an American court decision as to sentence.

Professor Gibbens makes the good point that defence counsel may well think twice before raising the XYY complement as a defence. Here is an inborn and permanent defect likely to have inborn and permanent disorders of behaviour. Who could blame a jury, if they knew of this, from handing down a conviction that would give indefinite protection to society.

I have written at length to try and clear the air (and my own mind) of the mass of disconnected evidence concerning this perhaps over-exploited abnormality. If my own interest has run away with me it might be excused on the grounds that Dr Sergovitch has handed me a priceless heritage: four randomly discovered newborns, XYY, for long term observation; they will be the subject of a detailed report when they all have reached two years of age. The oldest at present is 20 months, the youngest is 11 months old at the time of writing, December 1968.

Chapter XII
Intermediate States

Sex Chromosome Mosaics

While autosomal mosaicism seems to be uncommon in the living patient this is probably as much because abnormal stem lines, especially those that are monosomic, tend to die out as because mitotic mal-segregation in the zygote does not often happen. It seems that the frequency with which sex-chromosome mosaicism is found is a reflection of the fact that sex chromosome anomalies, even the deletions and monosomics, are not quite as lethal to the stem lines—as they are not as lethal to the individual—as anomalies of autosomal chromosomes. Almost every sex chromosome complement that has been found alone has been found in association with one or more cell lines with different chromosome constitution.

Mosaic individuals, presumably depending on the proportion of abnormal cells and perhaps on the timing of their appearance or dying-out, may exhibit either the full picture of the abnormality or a lesser degree of the disorder. If the abnormal cells are few in number or limited to an inaccessible or poorly growing tissue for culture purposes, the mosaicism may escape detection. The apparently XX male could be explained either by postulating that XY cells were too few to be detected, or by imagining that they had entirely died out—but after they had stimulated to medulla of the primitive gonad to develop as a testis, with the subsequent consequences that that differentiation entails.

Mosaic formation may not always be a bad thing. But for abnormal mitotic segregation things sometimes could be worse. Fig. 86 illustrates this. Suppose a female gamete is X but a fertilizing sperm bears no sex chromosome; the zygote will be XO. In the absence of further mal-divisions, all the body cells would be XO, and we would have a case of full-blown Turner's syndrome. But if another mitotic maldivision should follow this first error, a normal cell line could arise and modify the picture to the extent that the XX/XO female could pass for normal and even, as has happened, be fertile.

Mosaic Variants of Turner's Syndrome

One cannot here mention all the many and varied combinations of cell lines that could occur—or even that have been reported. A few examples must suffice.

The least degree of Turner's syndrome cytogenetically (though not the most common) is that in which there exists a normal cell line, XX, along with an Xx cell line. The patient XX/Xx would, because the

156

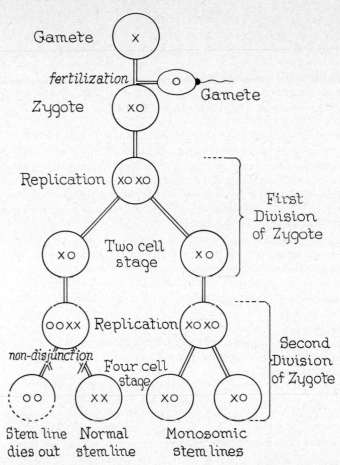

Fig. 86. Mosaicism Giving Partial Correction of the Abnormality. The Zygote is XO. The first division of the zygote gives two XO cells. At the next division, non-disjunction of one of those cells gives rise to OO and XX cells. If OO cells die out, a mosaic XX/XO is left. Such an individual may have modified Turner's syndrome, or may even be fertile.

short arms are present in all X chromosomes, be of normal stature but would have some degree of gonadal dysgenesis.

The mosaic XX/XX̄ has been discovered several times. The patients are short and have some of the somatic stigmata of Turner's syndrome along with gonadal dysgenesis.

The constitution XX/XO is the most common variant of Turner's syndrome, and as we have said, the expression of the disorder ranges from normality to the complete picture of Turner's syndrome with all its somatic deformities.

Several cases of triple stem-line mosaics have been recorded; XO/XX/XXX is an example. Three have Turner's syndrome, one is a normal woman and one a child with aganglionic megacolon.

Mosaicism in Klinefelter's Syndrome

Many variants on the XXY theme have been recorded. We can but mention a few—in order of departure from normality in cytogenic complement.

XY/XXY has a variable expression. It is the most common variant. There may be little or no abnormality; testicular atrophy and sterility are not invariable. There may or may not be mental retardation. Barr bodies in the buccal smear may not be found or may be found in small numbers depending on the representation of the two cell populations.

XY/XXXY has been reported several times. Klinefelter's syndrome in established form seems to be the result.

The first mosaic of XXY to be discovered was XX/XXY. Klinefelter's syndrome seems again to be the result, but in at least one case ambiguous genitalia and true hermaphroditism were found.

The triple stem-line mosaic XO/XY/XXY has been recorded. One of these patients is said, rather surprisingly to have had normal spermatogenesis. Another was sterile. A case of XY/XXY/XXXY mosaicism with rhematoid arthritis and reticulum cell sarcoma raises interesting speculation about the possible part played by autoimmune disease in chromosome anomaly and about the part played by chromosome anomaly in the aetiology of malignant disease.

One cannot leave the subject of mosaicism without a salute to the patient who achieved a mosaicism thus: XXXY/XXX/XXXY/XXXX/XXXXXY/XXXXX! No wonder he was mentally retarded.

Intersexuality and Pseudohermaphroditism

If it is difficult to define sexuality it is even more difficult to define intersex. If we take criteria of total sexuality to be of seven natures, chromosome constitution, gonad structure, morphology of external genitalia, morphology of internal ducts, hormonal status, sex of rearing and gender role, we can define intersexuality as a discrepancy between any of the first four. If discrepancy exists between either of the last two and any of the first four (they being in accord) we are into the subject of homosexuality, transexuality and transvestism. They hardly come within our purview in this book.

Concordancy of the first, second and fourth, but discordancy with the third, is exemplified by the adreno-genital syndrome with female pseudohermaphroditism and masculinization of the genitalia by excess androgenic hormones produced by other mechanisms than chromosome disorder.

Pseudohermaphroditism implies discordance between external genitalia and gonad structure. A male pseudohermaphrodite has testes but a female appearance. A female pseudohermaphrodite has ovaries but masculinized or ambiguous genitalia. A true hermaphrodite has both ovarian and testicular tissue, either as separate gonads or as a gonad that combines tissue of both types.

Within these terms of reference, Turner's syndrome scarcely qualifies as an intersex state. Although XO, there is no real discrepancy between our first four parameters. Klinefelter's syndrome is less easy to categorize, for there is an XX constitution albeit combined with Y to make XXY. Perhaps this cannot be called an intersexual state. Gonad structure, external genitalia and duct systems are concordant and the chromosome constitution not truly discrepant.

In the adreno-genital syndrome there may be intersexuality beyond doubt. One can have normal ovaries, normal chromosomes, XX, normal female ducts but ambiguous virilized genitalia. This is female pseudohermaphroditism because the adrenal glands unable, by autosomal recessive inborn metabolic error, to make hydrocortisone, turn out excessive androgens which affect the development of the external genitalia. The same effect of female pseudohermaphroditism can be produced by ingestion of androgenic hormones by a mother pregnant of a normal female foetus.

"Pure" gonadal dysgenesis XX is not of course an intersex state. The gonads were destined to be ovaries but suffered degeneration from other than genetic or chromosomal cause. The "Pure" gonadal dysgenesis XY, however, can be classified as intersex. There is discrepancy between the external genitalia that are female and the chromosomes that are XY. Admittedly the gonads should have developed as testes, but they did not; in spite of the XY chromosomes the genitalia continued to develop on female lines.

The Testicular Feminization Syndrome is an intersex; a male pseudohermaphroditism with an XY karyotype. The gonads are testes but the external genitalia, because of their unresponsiveness to androgenic steroid, failed to develop the appearance of maleness within the terms of reference that we laid down at the start of Chapter IX.

There are other varieties of intersex with pseudohermaphroditism but for the sake of clarity let us leave the matter there.

True Hermaphroditism

True hermaphrodities have both ovarian and testicular tissue. There may be "lateral hermaphrodites" where testicular tissue is on one side, ovarian on the other. They may be "bilateral" where both tissue are found together, combined, on both sides. They may be "unilateral", where only one gonad is found, and that again a combination.

The genitalia are usually ambiguous but the common phallic enlargement usually leads to their being classified at birth as males.

Nevertheless there is usually a vagina of sorts and variable degrees of Mullarian and Wolffian duct development. At puberty many of the patients show breast development and menstruation.

The chromosome complement is variable. Usually it is XX. The development of testicular tissue, even though combined with ovarian tissue, seems to imply, initially at least, an XY stem line. It seems likely that these embryos may have started as mosaics but with a subsequent elimination of the XY line. Some certainly are mosaics XX/XY, XX/XXYY, XX/XXY/XXYYY and other combinations.

Dissimilar "Identical" Twins

To complete our tale of the chromosome disorders one must make mention of this paradox. How could monzygotic twins be different, even in phenotypic sex? There is an explanation. Suppose, by non-disjunction of an XY zygote two stem lines were formed, XO and XYY. Then let us suppose that, after this non-disjunction, the embryo split to form a pair of monzygotic twins, each developing separately from these two stem lines, XO and XYY. A boy and girl monozygotic twins would result, entirely concordant in all respects but one; sex. The one would be XYY, with all that that may imply. The other would be a female, albeit with Turner's Syndrome. The same mechanism could account for "identical" twins discordant for mongolism. Such things have happened.

Chapter XIII
What Next?

In the first edition of this book I suggested certain lines of development in the future of cytogenetics and mentioned a number of questions to which answers are sadly lacking. In the three years that have passed since I last wrote this chapter those questions largely remain unanswered.

In spite of an enormous increase in the number of studies made we still are ignorant of the variations in the characteristics of normal human chromosomes, in the significance of any of the minor variations and of the frequency of even major structural re-arrangements. If the significance of, let us say, the YY constitution is to be known, we must know how many such are born and walk unnoticed in our midst. Large random surveys must be done even though the work entailed is tedious and costly.

We must know more of the effect of drugs and other agents on meiosis, mitosis, breaks, deletions and inversions. How harmful truly is, let us say, L.S.D? How risky really is a chest X-ray? How much does a pyelogram add to the risk of malsegregation at meiosis? What harm are we doing to future generations? Irene Uchida in a very recent study has noted a significant increase in the number of trisomic children born after maternal radiation exposure and concludes that mothers who have been exposed to abdominal radiological examination run, especially if they are older, an increased risk of producing non-disjunctional offspring.

In the not too distant future, indeed perhaps even now, we must worry about ionizing radiations on the chromosomes of astronauts; and they may be our children. I am prepared to bet that already our space travellers have had their gonads biopsied to observe if their meiosis at spermatogenesis is normal.

What are the effects of viruses in influencing chromosome re-arrangements? The effect of the virus of infective hepatitis has been noted by some to be apparently related to chromosome anomaly. It is true that this effect has been denied by others. Even such ubiquitous agents as the adenoviruses are suspect. It may, or may not be coincidence, that autoimmune thyroid disease is related to such virus infections. It may be coincidence that autoimmune thyroid disease is related to chromosome disorder; but it may not. There is more than a suspicion that leukaemia may be precipitated by virus infection in certain individuals who react abnormally to their infection. Is the increased incidence of leukaemia in mongolism related to immunological abnor-

161

mality: either in the way in which the mongol handles infections, or in the way he handles somatic mutations that are probably part and parcel of the lives of us all?

What is it that accounts for the weak familiality of even non-disjunction mongolism? It does not seem to be an innate difference alone. In our studies we could detect no difference whatever in the reproductive performance of mothers of mongols; no hint of an increased tendency to non-disjunction. Yet it is there, apparently. What then may be the factor to which they could be exposed that acts upon an undetected familial quality and produces non-disjunction? Why were the incidence figures from Bombay so different from those in Edinburgh? What was the unknown influence in Denver that so altered the incidence in the newborns in two hospitals at different times?

No doubt the time will come when refinements of technique will enable us to see morphological changes in chromosomes associated with disorders as small as gene mutations. Studies of phenotypic changes in chromosome disorders may tell us where to look. We are beginning tentatively to map the gene loci of the chromosomes. Is the gene locus of cystic fibrosis on the short arm of B5? Even though we know that some 60 genes are located on the X chromosome we do not know where their individual loci are. If one or two could be located studies of genetic linkage could lead to location of the others.

So many questions unanswered. What newly has been achieved or is on the brink of coming to fruition? Antenatal karyotpying is with us now. It can be done with good likelihood of success. One can already see its practical application if our thinking on the sanctity of foetal life and the dictates of the law allow those applications.

Animal oocytes have been fertilized in vitro, grown in culture as zygotes to a certain stage, scrutinized for karyotype and been implanted in the uterus, there to grow and fulfil the prognostications of the cytogeneticist. This could be applied to man. A zygote shown to be genetically undesirable could be discarded; only the good ones reserved for use.

"Crops" of ovarian follicles can be made to ripen at one time by the administration of pituitary follicle-stimulating hormones and an examination made of the chromosomes in the metaphase of the first meiotic division. Gonad biopsy after such stimulation could help us to counsel a woman as to her risk of non-disjunction.

There is a future, even a present, for biochemical study of cultured foetal cells. The cells of a foetus with the Lisch-Nyham uricacidaemia can be recognized after culture of cells exfoliated into the amniotic sac. Now it seems that the cells of a foetus destined to suffer cystic fibrosis may soon be identifiable by their development of metachromatic granules in tissue culture.

Where is all this leading? Is man on the brink of a new eugenics? Can he, should he, hand down a selected heritage to generations yet to come?

"Ah, my dear Watson, there we come to the realms of conjecture where the most logical mind may be at fault. Each may form his own hypothesis upon the present evidence, and yours is as likely to be correct as mine."

The Empty House
Arthur Conan Doyle

Some Recommended Reading

I must admit that I would be unable to quote chapter and verse for much of the information in this book. A great deal has been gleaned from conversations with my friends in the department of Anatomy of the University of Western Ontario and with Dr F. Sergovich of the Children's Psychiatric Research Institute here in London, Canada. For this knowledge I often cannot cite the original source. Nevertheless, most of the information will be found in amplified form in the writings listed below. I have found these articles and books particularly helpful, easy to understand or of special interest.

General Genetics and Cytogenetics
1. The Cell: Life Science Library. Time Incorporated, New York.
2. Genetics in Medicine: J. Thompson and M. Thompson. W. B. Saunders Co., Philadelphia and London, England.
3. Lectures in Medical Genetics: D. Yi-Yung Hsia. Year Book Medical Publishers, Inc., Chicago, U.S.A.
4. Human Developmental Genetics: D. Yi-Yung Hsia. Year Book Medical Publishers, Inc., Chicago, U.S.A.
5. Genetics for the Clinician: C. A. Clarke. Charles C. Thomas, Publisher, Springfield, Illinois, U.S.A.
6. Chromosomes in Medicine: J. L. Hammerton. Little Club Clinics in Developmental Medicine, No. 5. Heinemann Medical Books, Ltd., London, England.
7. Genetics in Medical Practice: M. Bartalos. J. B. Lippincott Company, Philadelphia, U.S.A. and Toronto, Canada.
8. Introduction to Genetics, a *Program for Self-Instruction*: McCraw-Hill Book Company, New York, San Francisco, Toronto, London.

Derminal Ridge Patterns
9. Finger Prints: Sir Francis Galton (reprinted 1965, with introduction by H. Cummins). Da Capo Press, New York.
10. Memorandum on Dermatoglyphic Nomenclature, vol. IV, No. 3 1968: L. S. Penrose. The National Foundation—March of Dimes, New York, U.S.A.
11. Fundamentals of Dermatoglyphics: R. C. Gibbs. Arch. Derm. 96: 721: 1967.
12. Dermatoglyphic Analysis as a Diagnostic Tool: M. Alter. Medicine 46: 35: 1966.
13. Unusual Dermatoglyphics Associated with Major Congenital Malformations: R. Achs et al., New. Eng. J. Med. 275: 1273: 1966.

Mongolism

14. Mongolism: C. E. Benda. Medical Aspects of Mental Retardation, Charles C. Thomas, 1965, Springfield, Illinois, U.S.A.
15. The Child with Mongolism: C. E. Benda. Grune and Stratton, 1960 New York.
    Author's note. I understand an entirely rewritten edition is in the press.
16. Mongolism (Commemoration of Dr John Haydon Langdon Down), Edited by G. E. W. Wolstenholme and Ruth Porter. J. A. Churchill, Ltd., London, England.
17. Medical Cytogenetics, Chap. 17: M. Bartalos, T. Baramki. The Williams and Wilkins Company, 1967 Baltimore, U.S.A.
18. The Use of Dermal Configurations in the Diagnosis of Mongolism: Normal Ford Walker, Paediatric Clinics of North America, 1958. W. B. Saunders Co., Philadelphia and London.

Other Autosomal Anomalies

19. Medical Cytogenetics, Chaps. 18, 19, 20: see 17 above.
20. Guide to Human Chromosome Defects, Vol. IV, No. 4, 1968: A. Redding and K. Hirschorn. The National Foundation—March of Dimes, New York, U.S.A.
21. Syndrome of Partial Deletion of Long Arm of Chromosome 18: J. Insley: Arch, Dis. Child. 42: 140: 1967.
22. Le Syndrome du Cri du Chat: J. DeGrouchy et al. Annals de Genetique, 7: 13: 1964.
23. Autosomal Monosmy in Man: M. Al-Aish et al. New Eng. J. Med. 227: 777: 1967.

Incidence of Chromosome Anomalies

24. Chromosome Anomalies as a Cause of Spontaneous Abortion: D. H. Carr. Amer. J. Obst., Gynec. 97: 283: 1967.
25. Anatomic Findings in Human Abortions of Known Chromosomal Constitution: R. P. Singh and D. H. Carr. Obstetrics and Gynecology 29: 806: 1967.
26. Chromosome After Oral Contraceptives, D. H. Carr: Lancet, 2: 830: 1967.
27. Sex Chromosome Abnormalities in Newborn babies: N. Maclean et al. Lancet, 1: 286: 1964.
28. Human Population Cytogenetics: W. M. Court Brown 1967. North Holland Publishing Company, Amsterdam, Netherlands, and John Wiley and Sons Inc., New York.

Sex Chromosomes and Sex Chromosome Anomalies

29. Medical Cytogenetics, Chaps. 4–15: See 17 above.
30. Intersexuality: C. Overzier. Academic Press, London and New York.
31. Classification of Intersexuality: C. Overzier. Triangle, 8; 32–40: 1967.
32. XO Syndrome Review: Editorial Comment. Clinical Paediatrics, 6: 130: 67.
33. Criminal Behaviour and the Y chromosome: Editorial Comment, Brit. Med. J., 1: 64: 1967.
34. XYY Constitution in Prepubertal Child: J. Cowie, J. Kahn. Brit. Med. J., 1: 748: 68.
35. Behaviour Disorders and Pattern of Crime among XYY Males Identified at a Maximum Security Hospital: W. H. Price, P. B. Whatmore. Brit. Med. J., 1: 533: 67.
36. Heredity and Responsibility: W. M. Court Brown. New Scientist, 31 Oct.: 235: 1968.
37. Genetics and Ethics: T. C. N. Gibbens. New Scientist, 31 Oct.: 236: 1968.
38. Sex Chromosomes and Aberrant Behaviour: Editorial Comment. Medical-Moral Newsletter Vol. V: 9: Nov. 1968.

For general knowledge of this whole subject I would recommend, above all others listed: 2, 3, 6, 8, 17.

Index